PHARMACY TECHNICIAN CERTIFIED BOARD PREP: CROSSWORD PUZZLES AND WORD SEARCH

Pharmacy Technician Certified Board Prep: Crossword Puzzles and Word Search

Anne Nguyen

For more information visit, **www.ptcbprep.com**.

This book was printed in the United States of America.

Rev. date: 03/13/2014

To order additional copies of this book, contact:
Xlibris LLC
1-888-795-4274
www.Xlibris.com
Orders@Xlibris.com
540216

Contents

ANSWERS TO
CROSSWORD PUZZLES
AND
WORD SEARCH

To my family for the time they sacrificed so that this book would become a reality. Especially to my parents, who have nourished my body with food and challenged my brain academically until the end of time.

I am grateful to my family, especially my oldest sister, Kim Pham, who has motivated and encouraged me to fulfill a lifelong dream.

To my brother and all my sisters for their continuous support of my career through the years, and to my mentors and advisors, whose vision provided education and motivation that encouraged my professional growth and challenged me to be an innovator.

Preface

The objective of this crossword puzzle book is to prepare students for their future as Pharmacy Technician and to have a success in taking the national certified pharmacy board exam. A pharmacy technician career is very demanding and to become a national certified pharmacy technician, one must be prepared because the cost of the exam is expensive and will continue to rise. All students must review and prepare for this board exam. There are different study techniques that can be employed, including flash cards, practice tests, and games, such as crossword puzzles. It is important to select the right method to study for the board exam. Whichever methods students select will have an impact on the outcome of the exam. These crosswords puzzles can help students to memorize and recognize the answer since the board exam is mainly multiple choices.

The national board exam consists of many mixed categories which can be one of the followings:

1. 80 % math and 20 % drugs
2. 80 % retail and 20 % hospital
3. 70 % hospital and 30 % math
4. 75 % retail and 25 % math
5. 90 % top 300 drugs and 10 % math

This national board exam is not simple to pass unless students have mastered their drugs knowledge as well as other subjects. To increase the success in passing the board exam the first time, one must use these crossword or word search methodology to study and attend the preparation classes. This book consists mainly of brand names and generic names of the top 300 hundred drugs with their drug classifications. Students who use crossword puzzles can retain in memory these drug names much better and will have a higher chance of passing the exam. It is not easy to shuffle these 300 hundred brand names and generic drugs names. Study has shown that our brain can only take in less than 40 percent each day.

Studying is a very time-consuming process. It takes time for our brain to digest, store, and convert read items into long-term memories. Crossword puzzles and word searches are, by far, the most effective method of learning for most students. It can help student build confidence when it is time to take the exam.

The national certified board of pharmacy exam contains questions that are for pretrial purposes and will not be scored. Students will not know which questions are scored and which are not. It is best to attempt to answer every question. Students who use this textbook and attend the preparation classes will have greater chances of passing the board exam.

About the Author

Anne Nguyen is a pharmacist in the state of Texas with over twenty years of experience in retail, hospital, and mail order combined. She graduated as cum laude with a bachelor of science in pharmacy from the College of Pharmacy at Southwestern Oklahoma State University, Weatherford, Oklahoma, in 1992 and a doctor of pharmacy from Idaho State University, Pocatello, Idaho, in 2010.

Ms. Nguyen held positions as a clinical pharmacist at the Dallas Medical Center and a remote order entry pharmacist for most of North Texas hospitals and retail pharmacies. She received a Distinguished Service Award in the North Texas Region of Eckerd Pharmacy in 1999. Her Eckerd Drugstore was a training store for all newly hired pharmacists and student interns.

Ms. Nguyen serves as a pharmacist preceptor for the state of Texas since 1993. She is a certified immunizer from AphA, ACLS, and BLS. She is a certified instructor of IV certification classes through University of Houston College of Pharmacy.

When she is not teaching one-on-one, she is a coauthor of several books including *PTCB Comprehensive Review Manual* and *1,001 PTCB Exam Review Questions*.

She is currently one of a few pioneer pharmacists working as remote order entry from home. Ms. Nguyen also works as a clinical coordinator pharmacist at the Dallas Medical Center hospital, PRN floater for Costco Drugstore, and PRN staff at Super Value Drugstore. With her well-rounded experience in this pharmaceutical industry, she has established a well network of connections with most retail drugstores and hospitals in the Dallas and Fort Worth area.

Foreword

This puzzle publication is a significant and unique addition to pharmacy references. It should be considered for anyone with or without pharmacy experience who wants to become a nationally certified pharmacy technician. I am pleased that it is a very helpful and fun study technique by far. I recommend this to be on every current and aspiring student's bookshelf or backpack.

Crosswords and word search puzzles are designed exercises to help students master memorization skills. It can be very useful in identifying areas of understanding as well as lack of comprehension and other areas of weakness. Students will be able to apply what they learn into this workbook. When students have difficulty with crossword puzzles, it will prompt them to research the correct answers. Crossword puzzles have shown to be very successful in helping students retain their learning materials and have a positive outcome in the exam. Often these crossword puzzles and word searches are perceived as a recreational activity. Therefore, students enjoy them.

This workbook contains crossword puzzles and word searches of more than 40 different types of category of medications. It also covers the top three hundred most common drugs. They are the following subjects:

- Pharmacy Technician Duties
- Common Pharmacy References
- Pharmacy Law Review
- Pharmacy Health Insurance Review
- Different Types of Vaccines
- Different Types of Dosage Forms
- Different Routes of Administration
- Different Sites of Practices (Retail, Hospital, Mail Order, Home Health)
- Antibiotics (Penicillins, Cephalosporins, Quinolones, Sulfa Drugs, and Other Antibiotics)
- Antihypertensive Medications (Angiotensin Converting Enzyme Inhibitors, Calcium Blockers, Beta-Blockers, Antiarrhythmics)

- Antidepressants
- Antidotes
- Antihistamines
- Common Respiratory Medications
- Diabetic Medications and Supplies
- Common Drugs Used in Blood Transfusion
- Common Over-the-Counter Medications
- Anti-Parkinson's Medications
- Antifungal Medications
- Common Heartburn Medications
- Pain Medications (Narcotics and Nonnarcotics)
- Osteoporosis Medications
- Benzodiazepine Medications
- Antihyperlipidemic Medications
- Antiarrhythmic Medications
- Anticancer Medications
- Human Immunodeficiency Virus (HIV) Medications
- Urinary Incontinence Medications
- Topical Steroids
- Topical Acne Medications
- Ear Drop Medications
- Common Ophthalmic Medications
- Common Medications Used in Dialysis
- Common Drugs that Interact with Grapefruit Juice
- Common Drugs Used in Palliative Care for Comfort Measure
- Common Drugs with Black Box Warnings
- Common Drugs Available in Orally Disintegrating Tablet Forms
- Common Drugs Need to be Avoided After Gastric Bypass
- Cytochrome Enzyme Inhibitors
- Cytochrome Enzyme Inducers
- Intravenous Medications that Require In-Line Filters
- Common Medications that Cannot Be Crushed

This book is definitely a valuable resource alongside the *Pharmacy Technician Certified Board Preparation: Comprehensive Review Manual* for all students who want to pass the pharmacy board exam the first time. It would be a fun way to retain pharmacy knowledge.

Angiotensin Converting Enzyme (ACE) Inhibitors

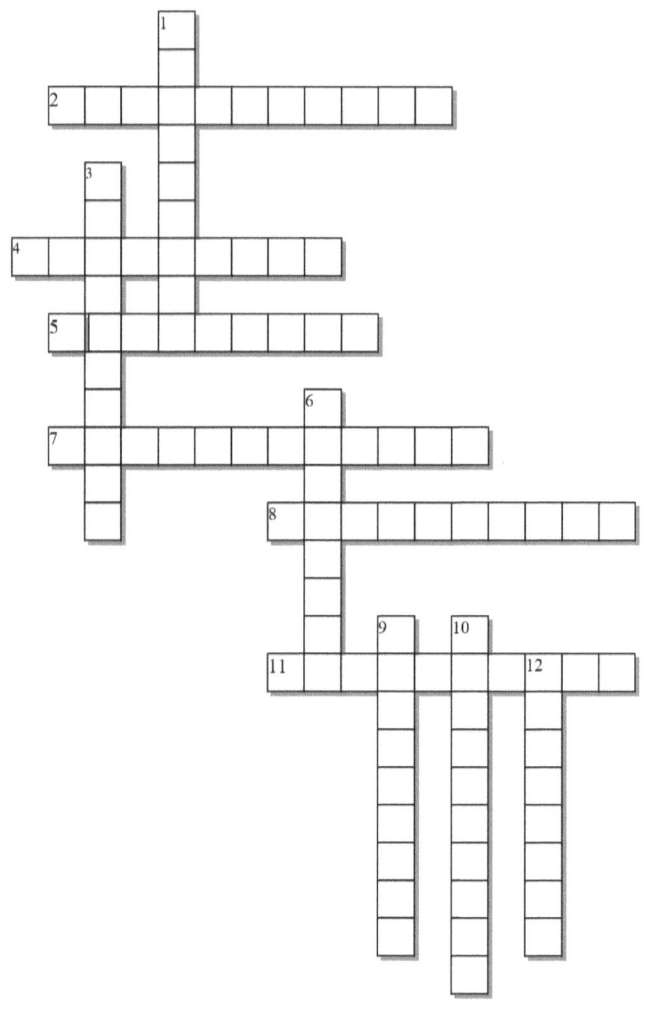

Across:

2. Generic name for Aceon®
4. Brand name for enalapril-HCT
5. Generic name for Vasotec®
7. Generic name for Mavik®
8. Generic name for Monopril®

11. Generic name for Lotensin®

Down:

1. Generic name for Accupril®
3. Generic name for Zestril®
6. Brand name for captopril-HCT
9. Generic name for Capoten®
10. Brand name for lisinopril-HCTZ

12. Generic name for Altace®

Antiarrhythmic Medications

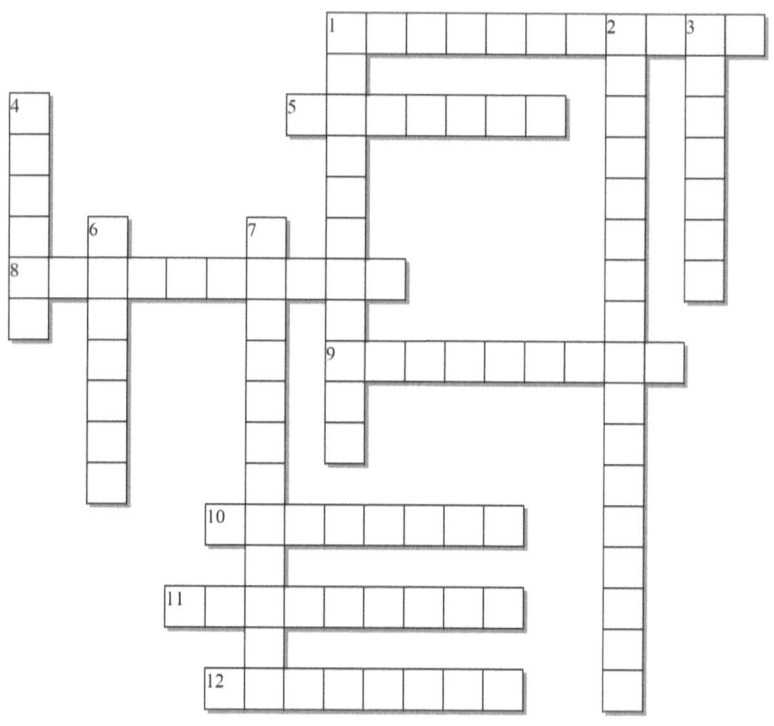

Across:

1 - Generic name for Rythmol®

5 - Brand name for ibutilide

8 - Generic name for Cordarone®

9 - Generic name for Xylocaine®

10 - Brand name for flecainide

11 - Generic name for Quinaglute®

12 - Brand name for sotalol

Down:

1 - Generic name for Inderal®

2 - Antiarrhythmic medications help the heart to maintain its normal rhythm, which is also known as NSR (what does this abbreviation stand for?)

3 - Brand name for disopyramide

4 - Brand name for dronedarone

6 - Trade name for dofetilide

7 - Generic name for Procanbid®

Antibiotics

```
R I V O L C Y C A M P I C I L L I N D R V D
T O B R A M Y C I N O I D D D O X C E T A K
N O F L O X A C I N N G P L O R G E N E N X
I M Q S Z Z X C I P R O E E X A K F I T C F
L N N I X A I B F Z S V N P Y C Z A L R O X
L I C B Q B B N O A O I I M C A I D C A M O
I C E A U R I S A F L N W H Y R T R Y C Y L
C E F C Z Z Y M L C Y S J C L B H O C Y C E
I F A T E N U O Y S E R Y C I E R X Y C I V
N I C R V U X C A Y L F Y Z N F O I X L N A
E V L I Q A O N W S W W E C E F M L O I U B
P X O M C N U X O X E L F E K C A R D N B D
M Y R I I X K O F C E F T R I A X O N E D S
S A N M O X I F L O X A C I N F C P Q G I U
```

acyclovir
Bactrim®
cefaclor
Cipro®
Doxycyline
Keflex®
Macrobid®
Ofloxacin
Tetracycline
Vancomycin
Zosyn®

ampicillin
Biaxin®
Cefadroxil
Cubicin®
Eryc®
Levofloxacin
Minocycline
Omnicef®
Tobramycin
Zinacef®

Avelox®
Ceftriaxone
Doxycycline
Gentamicin
Loracarbef
Moxifloxacin
Penicillin
Unasyn®
Zithromax®

Anticancer Medications

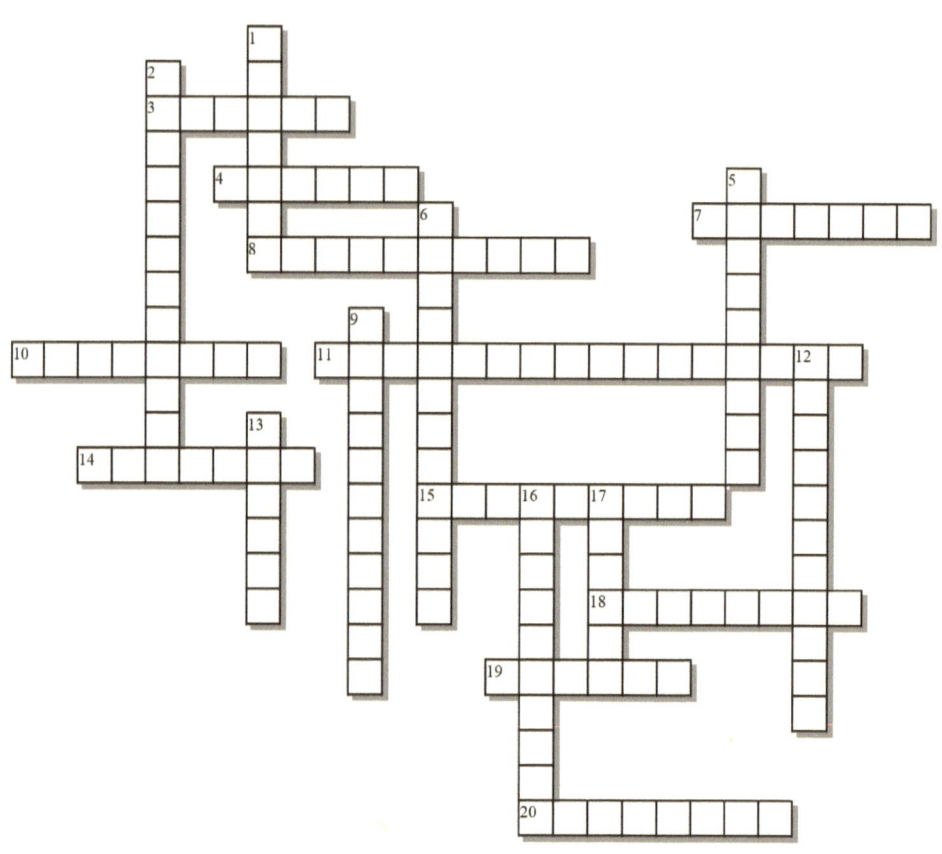

Across:

3 - Trade name for leuprolide

4 - Brand name for capecitabine

7 - Brand name for imatinib

8 - Generic name for Emend®

10 - Trade name for tamoxifen citrate

11 - Generic name for Cytoxan®

14 - Brand name for goserelin

15 - Generic name for Alkeran®

18 - Brand name for exemestane

19 - Trade name for letrozole

20 - Brand name for chlorambucil

Down:

1 - Brand name for erlotinib

2 - Generic name for Efudex®

5 - Generic name for Eulexin®

6 - Generic name for Casodex®

9 - Generic name for Hydrea®

12 - Generic name for Adriamycin®

13 - Brand name for gemcitabine

16 - Brand name for mercaptopurine

17 - Brand name for imiquimod

Antidepressant Medications

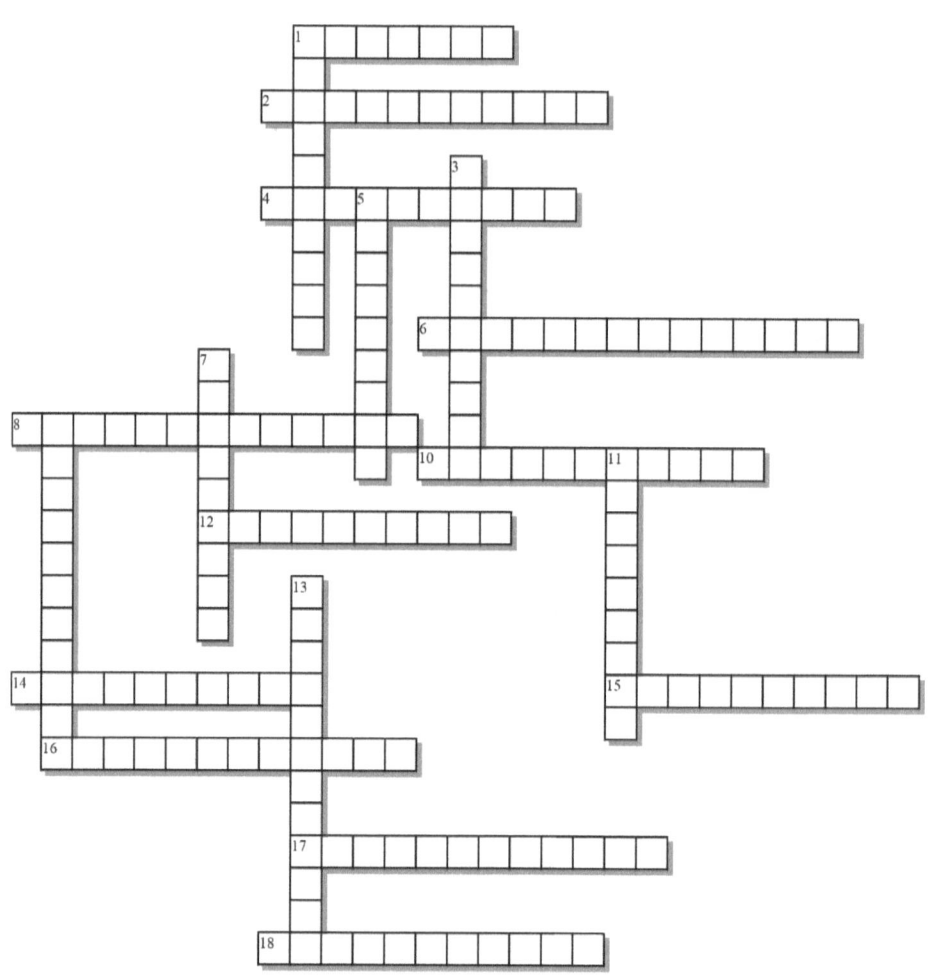

Across:

1 - Generic for Sinequan®
2 - Generic for Luvox®
4 - Generic for Zoloft®
6 - Generic for Pristiq®
8 - Generic for Elavil®
10 - Generic for Norpramin®
12 - Generic for Paxil®
14 - Generic for Celexa®
15 - Generic for Serzone®
16 - Generic for Lexapro®
17 - Generic for Ludiomil®
18 - Generic for Effexor®

Down:

1 - Generic for Cymbalta®
3 - Generic for Prozac®
5 - Generic for Desyrel®
7 - Generic for Wellbutrin®
9 - Generic for Remeron®
11 - Generic for Asendin®
13 - Generic for Anafranil®

Anti-Drug Category

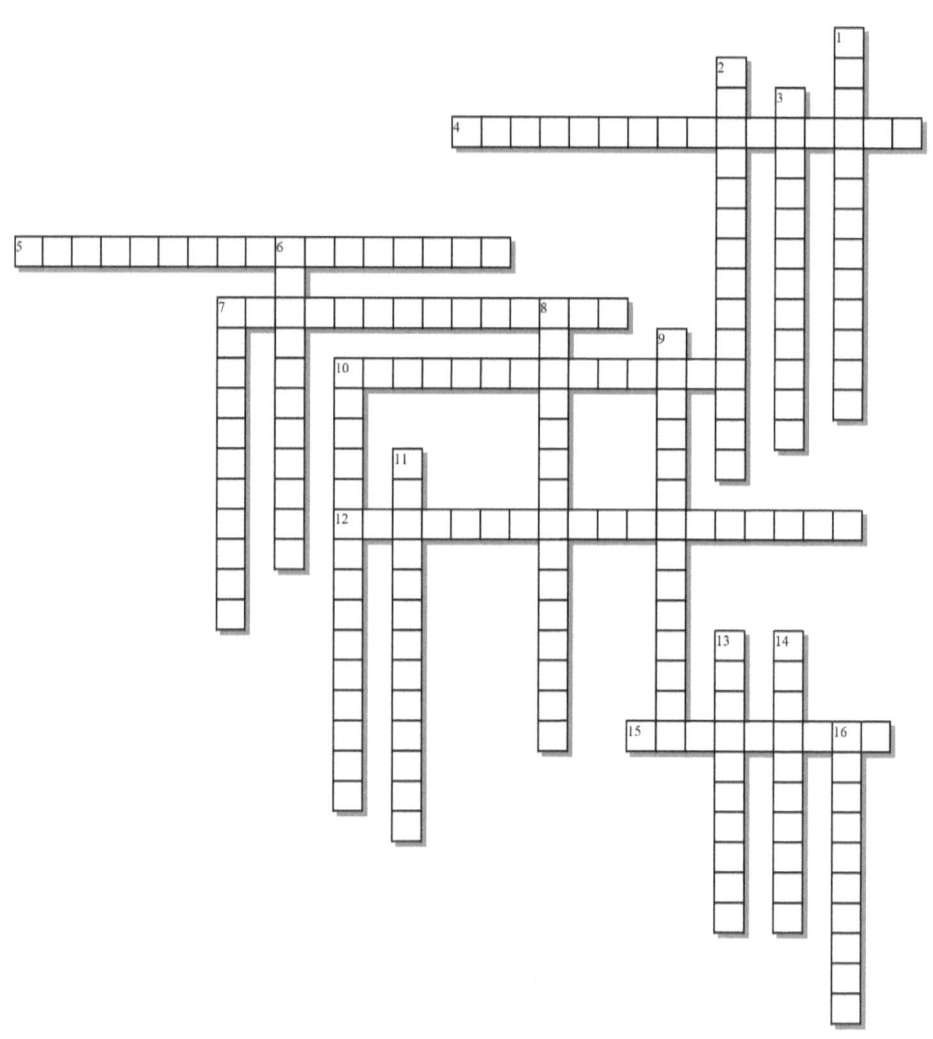

Across:

4 - This group of drugs treats high blood pressure

5 - This group of drugs treats inflammation and pain

7 - This group of drugs treats seizures

10 - A group of drugs that treats allergies

12 - This group of drugs is used in lowering high cholesterol

15 - This group of drugs treats viral infection

Down:

1 - This group of drugs treats psychological disorders

2 - Another name for anticancer drugs

3 - This group of drugs is used in relieving itching or rash

6 - This group of drugs helps in reducing fever

7 - This group of drugs treats cough

8 - This group of drugs treats ADHD

9 - This group of drugs treats depression

10 - This group of drugs slows heartbeat

11 - This group of drugs treats abdominal spasms

13 - A group of drugs that treats nausea

14 - This group of drugs treats bacterial infection

16 - This group of drugs treats fungal infection

Antifungal Medications

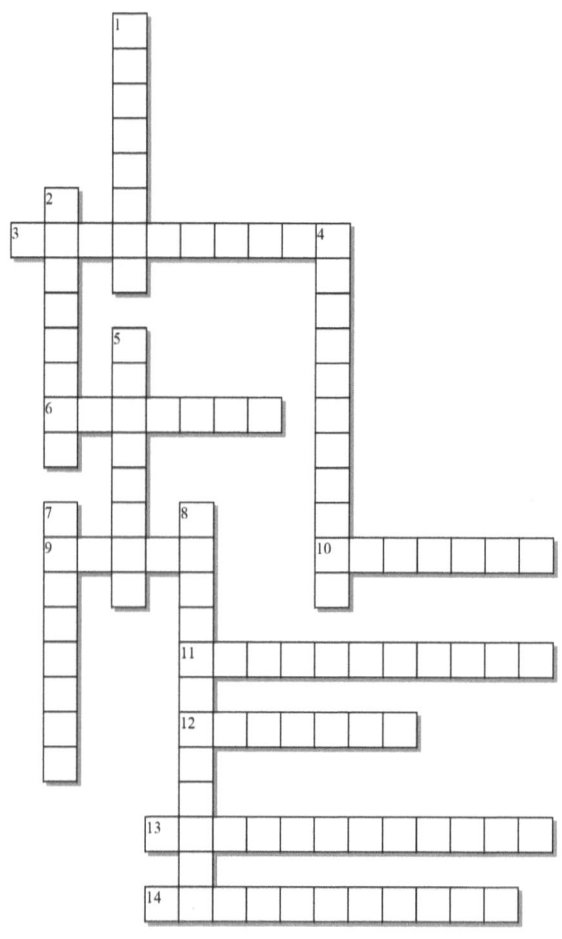

Across:

3 - Brand name for clotrimazole, available as OTC, which is used for jock itch

6 - Name the most common yeast infection

9 - Antifungal medications are used in treating _____ infection (please fill in the blank)

10 - Brand name for terbinafine

11 - Generic name for the injectable antifungal Cancidas®

12 - This brand-name medication is available as shampoo, has generic name of ketoconazole

13 - Generic name for Vfend®

14 - This generic medication is also available in 250 mg tablet form

Down:

1 - Name a type of fungal infection that appears on the surface of the skin with a ring around it

2 - Name a type of fungal infection where itching red rash appears in the groin area

4 - Generic name for Diflucan®

5 - Brand name for miconazole

7 - Brand name for micafungin

8 - Generic name for Sporanox®

Antihistamines

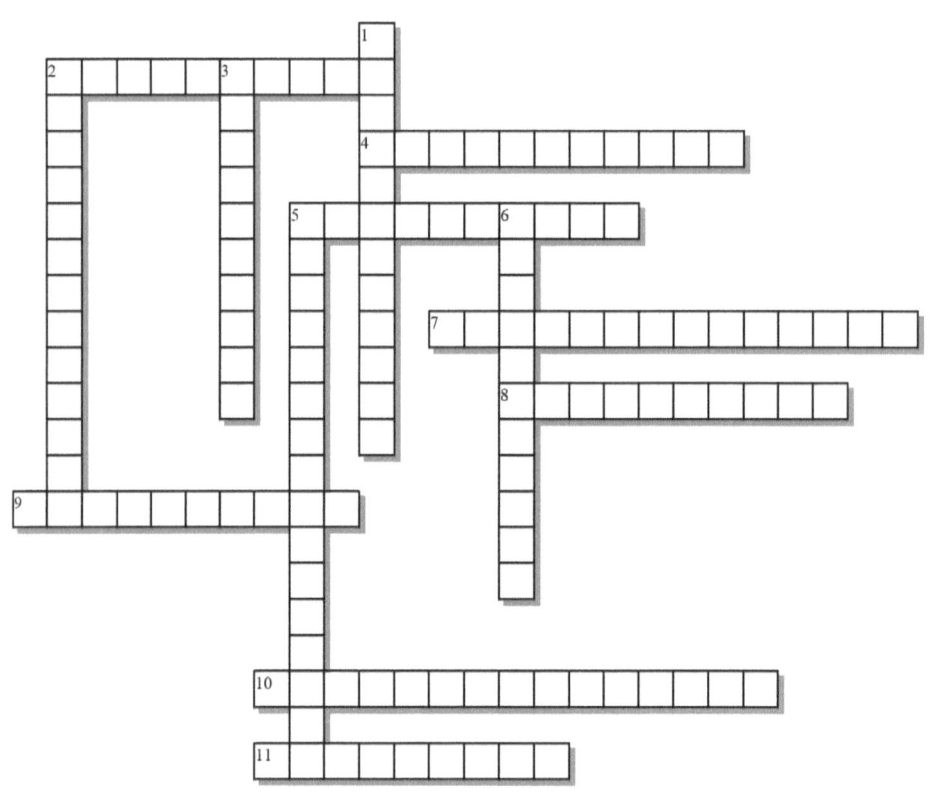

Across:

2 - Generic name for Unisom®

4 - Generic name for Patanol® eyedrops

5 - Generic name for Tavist-1®

7 - Generic name for Periactin®

8 - Generic name for Claritin®

9 - Generic name for Zyrtec®

10 - Generic name for Benadryl®

11 - Generic name for Antivert®

Down:

1 - Generic name for Allegra®

2 - Generic name for Clarinex®

3 - Generic name for Astelin®

5 - Generic name for Chlor-Trimeton®

6 - Name the main ingredient in Actifed®

Antihyperlipidemic Medications

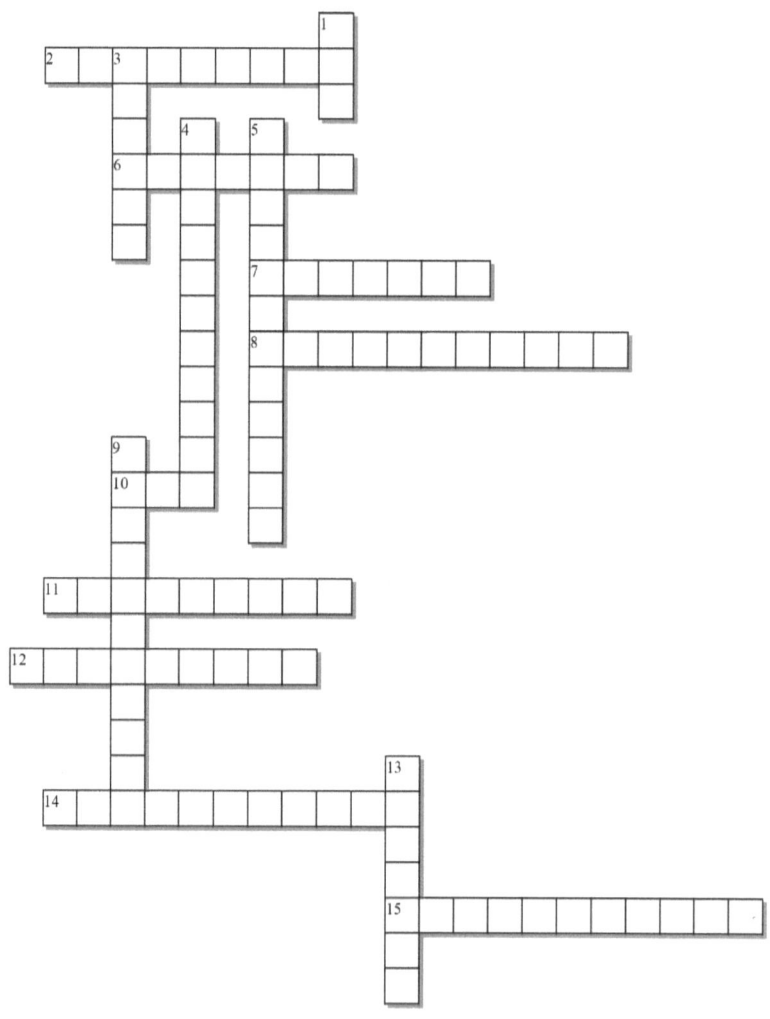

Across:

2 - Generic name for Colestid®

6 - Brand name for rosuvastatin

7 - Brand name for ezetimibe and simvastatin

8 - Generic name for Zocor®

10 - The abbreviation for low-density lipoprotein, often called bad cholesterol

11 - Brand name for pravastatin

12 - Generic name for Zetia®

14 - Generic name for TriCor®

15 - Generic name for Welchol®

Down:

1 - The abbreviation for high-density lipoprotein, this lab value often called good cholesterol

3 - Another brand name for omega-3 fatty acids

4 - Generic name for Lopid®

5 - Generic name for Lipitor®

9 - Generic name for Lescol®

13 - Trade name for lovastatin

Anti-Parkinson's Medications

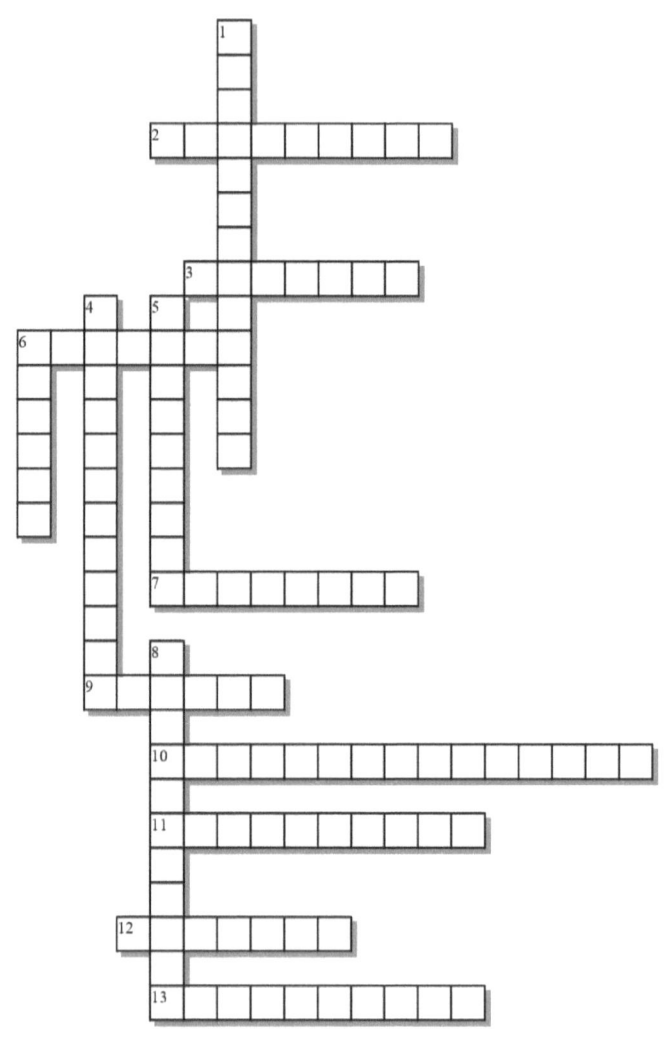

Across:

2 - Brand name for amantadine

3 - Brand name for carbidopa/ levodopa

6 - Trade name for rasagiline

7 - Brand name for selegiline

9 - This brand-name medication is available in patch dosage form and has the generic name of rivastigmine

10 - The only medication used in treating Parkinson's that is available in an oral disintegrating tablet form

11 - Generic name for Requip®

12 - Brand name for pramipexole

13 - Generic name for Comtan®

Down:

1 - Generic name for Parlodel®

4 - Generic name for Exelon®

5 - Generic name for Permax®

6 - Trade name for trihexyphenidyl

8 - Generic name for Cogentin®

Attention-Deficit/Hyperactivity Disorder Medications

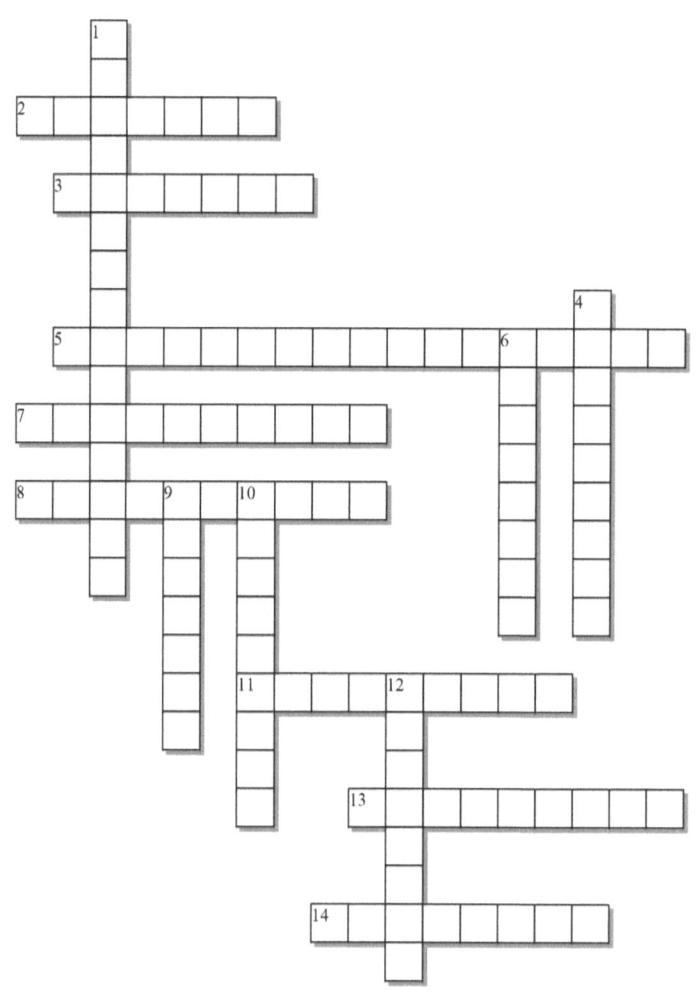

Across:

2 - Brand name for this long-acting guanfacine

3 - Brand name for lisdexamfetamine

5 - Generic name for Dexedrine®

7 - All ADHD medications are considered as _____

8 - Generic name for Tenex®, also used for attention deficit disorder

11 - This brand name for dextroamphetamine is available in capsule form

13 - Brand name for atomoxetine

14 - Brand name for methylphenidate that is available in strengths 18 mg, 27 mg, 36 mg, and 54 mg

Down:

1 - Generic name for Ritalin®

4 - Brand name for methylphenidate long-acting capsule

6 - Brand name for amphetamine capsule

9 - Brand name for this short-acting dextro isomer methylphenidate

10 - Generic name for Catapres®

12 - Brand name for this methylphenidate transdermal patch

Benzodiazepine Medications

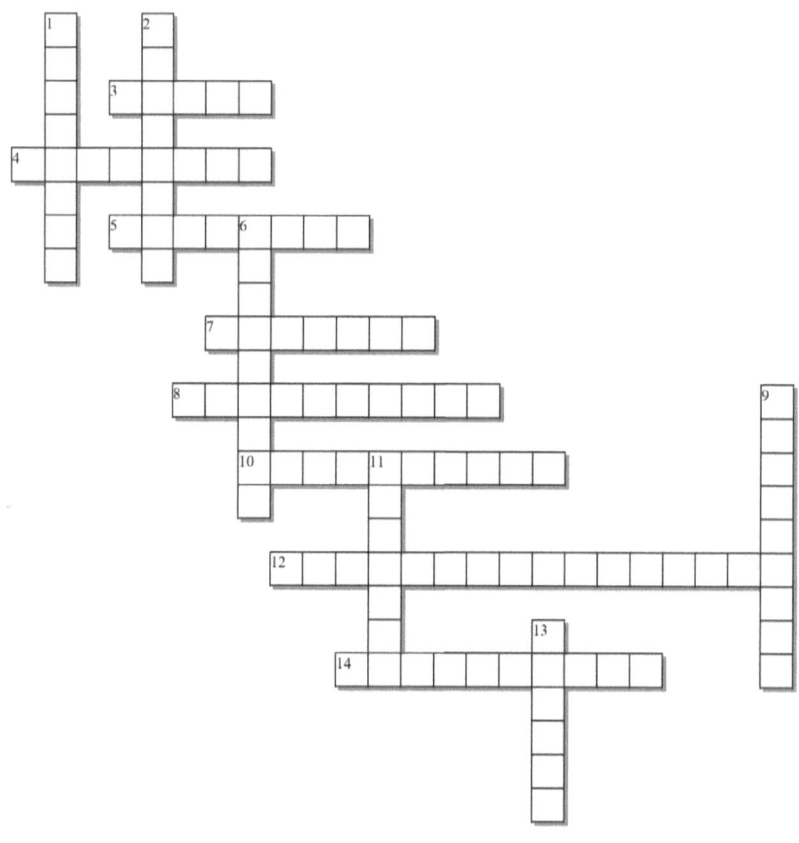

Across:

3 - Trade name for quazepam

4 - Brand name for temazepam

5 - Generic name for Valium®

7 - Trade name for triazolam

8 - What is the most common side effect of all benzodiazepines?

10 - Generic name for Xanax®

12 - Generic name for Librium®

14 - Generic name for Dorax®

Down:

1 - Generic name for Serax®

2 - Trade name for clonazepam

6 - Generic name for Prosom®

9 - Generic name for Ativan®

11 - It is recommended not to drink _____ with these medications because it can enhance the drowsiness

13 - Trade name for midazolam

Beta-Blockers Medications

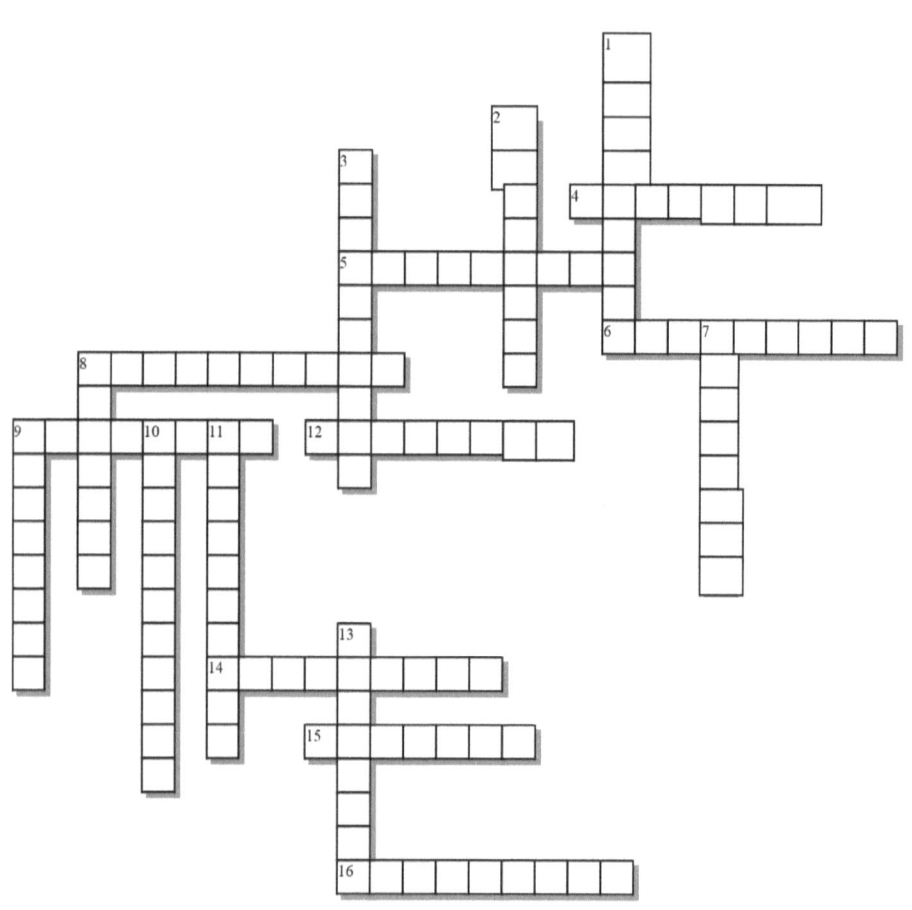

Across:

4 - Generic name for Timoptic®

5 - Generic name for Kerlone®

6 - Generic name for Ocupress®

8 - Generic name for Zebeta®

9 - Brand name for sotalol

12 - Brand name for metoprolol succinate

14 - Trade name for metoprolol tartrate

15 - Trade name for nadolol

16 - Another brand name for labetalol, starts with letter *N*

Down:

1 - Trade name for esmolol

2 - Generic name for Visken®

3 - Generic name for Sectral®

7 - Brand name for labetalol, starts with letter *T*

8 - Brand name for levobunolol

9 - Brand name for nebivolol

10 - Generic name for Inderal®

11 - Generic name for Coreg®

13 - Brand name for atenolol

Calcium Channel Blockers

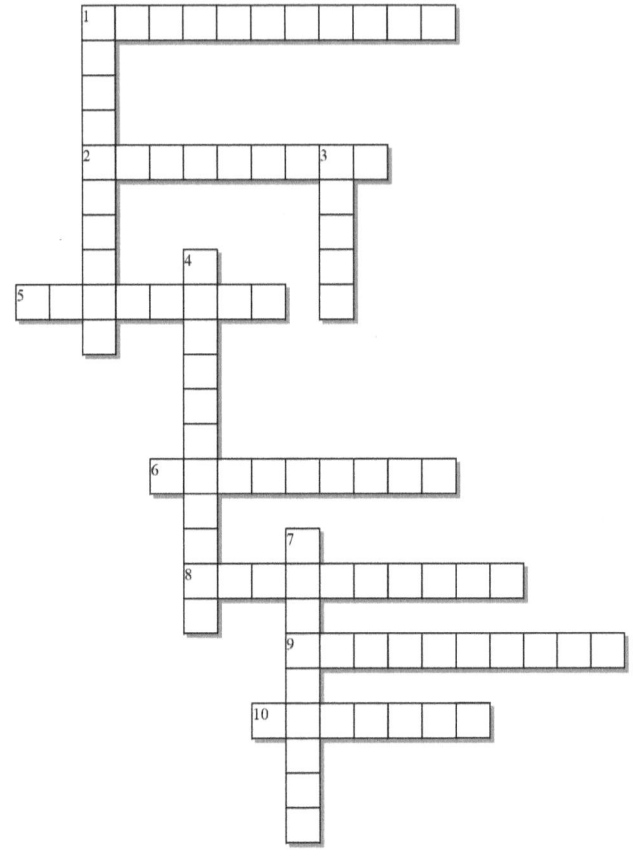

Across:

1 - Generic name for Cardene®

2 - Generic name for Cardizem®

5 - Brand name for isradipine

6 - These calcium channel blockers are used in treating ____ ____ pressure

8 - Generic name for Procardia®

9 - Generic name for Norvasc®

10 - This brand-name medication is also available as an injectable, used widely in every hospital as a drip

Down:

1 - Generic name for Nimotop®

3 - Most common side effects for calcium channel blockers

4 - Generic name for Sular®

7 - Generic name for Calan SR®

Central Nervous System Medications

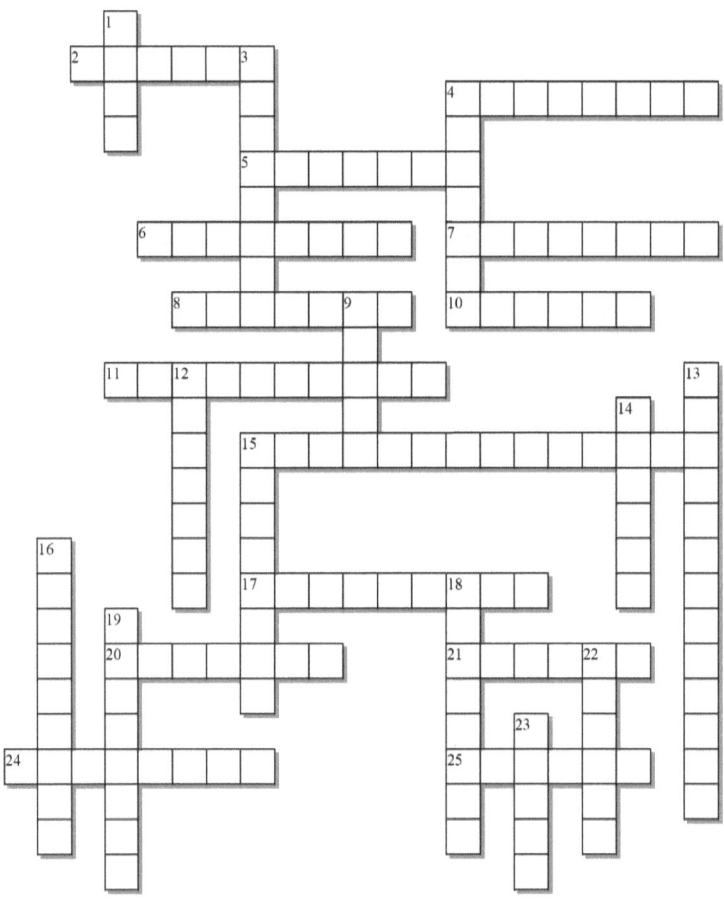

Across:

2. Brand name for sertraline

4. Brand name for phenytoin

5. Brand name for ramelteon

6. Brand name for hydroxyzine pamoate

7. Brand name for temazepam

8. Brand name for flurazepam

10. Brand name for pregabalin

11. Brand name for bupropion

15. A hypnotic medication

17. Brand name for gabapentin

21. Brand name for lorazepam

24. Brand name for morphine sulfate ER

25. Brand name for amitriptyline

Down:

1. Brand name for carisoprodol

3. Brand name for carbamazepine

4. Brand name for meperidine

9. Brand name for hydrocodone/ APAP

12. Brand name for eszopiclone

13. Anti-seizure drug (has the abbreviation of Pb)

14. Brand name for diazepam

15. Brand name for benztropine

16. Brand name for fentanyl

18. Brand name for clorazepate

19. Brand name for clonazepam

22. Brand name for zolpidem

23. Brand name for alprazolam

Cephalosporin Antibiotics

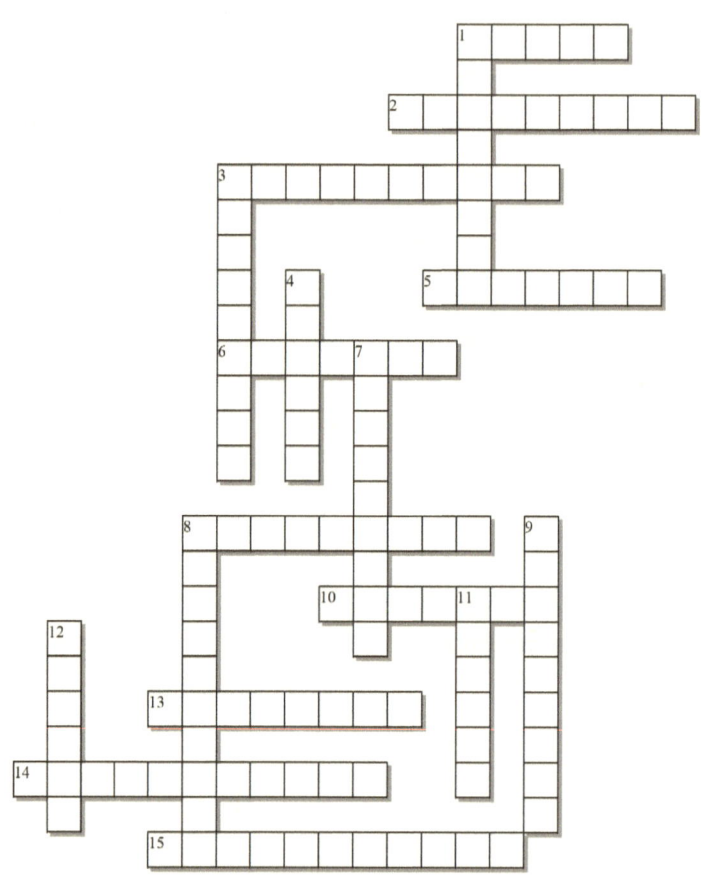

Across:

1 - Trade name for ceftibuten

2 - Generic name for Mefoxin®

3 - Generic name for Duricef®

5 - Trade name for cefoperazone

6 - Trade name for cefdinir

8 - Generic name for Ancef®

10 - Trade name for ceftazidime

13 - Brand name for cefepime

14 - Generic name for Rocephin®

15 - Generic name for Teflaro®

Down:

1 - Generic name for Suprax®

3 - Generic name for Cefzil®

4 - Brand name for cefpodoxime

7 - Generic name for Ceftin®

8 - Generic name for Claforan®

9 - Generic name for Cefotan®

11 - Brand name for cefaclor

12 - Brand name for cephalexin

Common Antidotes

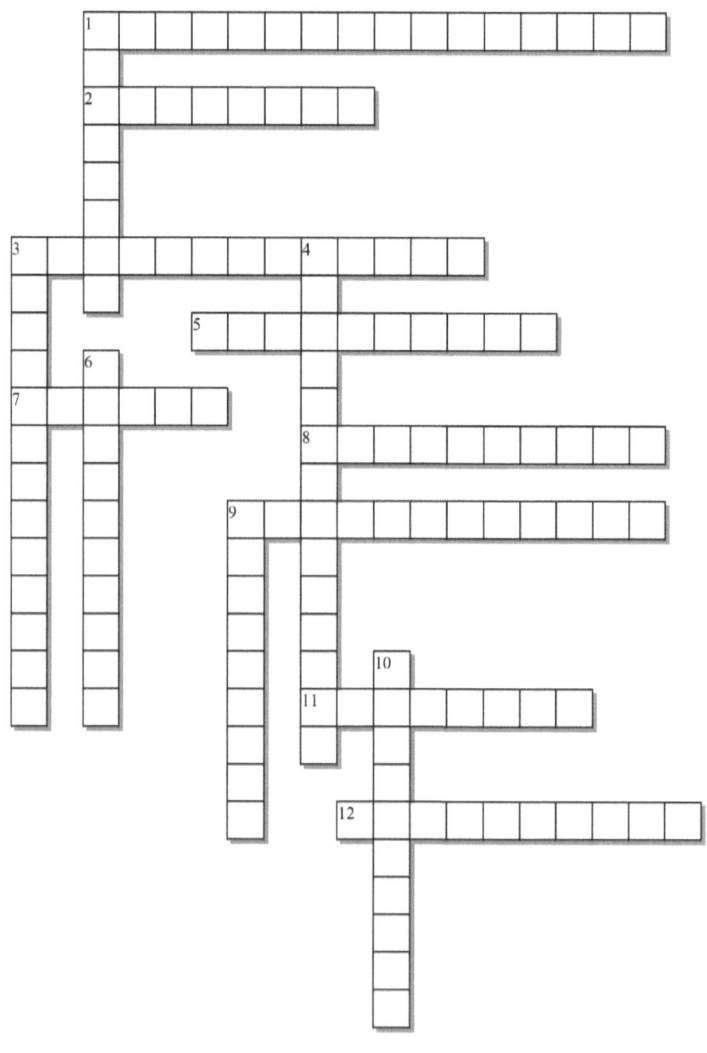

Across:

1. Used to treat drug overdose in insulin

2. Used to treat drug overdose in beta-blockers

3. Used to treat drug overdose in copper

5. Used to treat drug overdose in ethylene glycol

7. Used to treat drug overdose in carbon monoxide

8. Used to treat drug overdose in methotrexate

9. Used to treat drug overdose in warfarin

11. Used to treat drug overdose in opioids

12. Used to treat drug overdose in potassium

Down:

1. Used to treat drug overdose in digoxin

3. Used to treat drug overdose in anticholinergics

4. Used to treat drug overdose in acetaminophen

6. Used to treat drug overdose in isoniazid

9. Used to treat drug overdose in heparin

10. Used to treat drug overdose in benzodiazepines

Common Drugs Available in Orally Disintegrating Tablet Forms

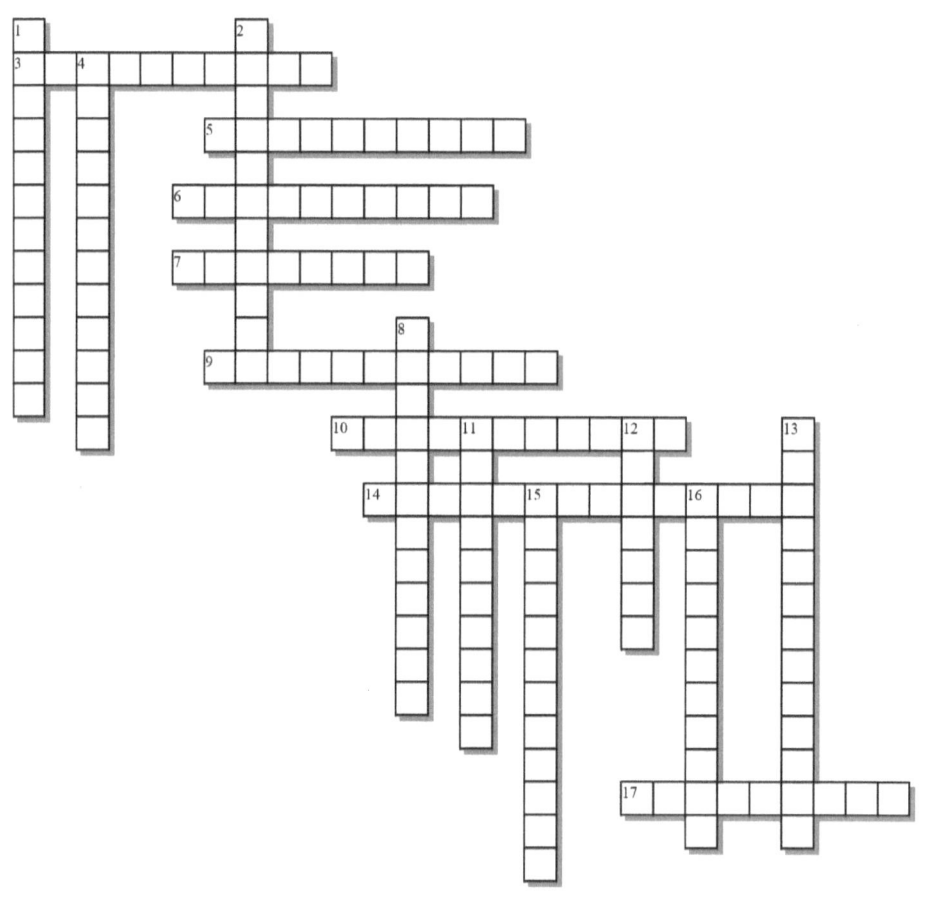

Across:

3 - An orally disintegrating tablet for FazaClo®

5 - An orally disintegrating tablet for Staxyn®

6 - Generic name for Claritin®

7 - Orally disintegrating tablet for phentermine

9 - Generic name for Zofran®

10 - Generic name for Symax®

14 - Generic name for Metozolv® or Reglan®

17 - Generic name for Aricept®

Down:

1 - Generic name for Zomig®

2 - Generic name for Maxalt®

4 - Generic name for Abilify®

8 - Generic name for Allegra®

11 - Generic name for Klonopin®

12 - An orally disintegrating tablet for alprazolam

13 - Generic name for Tylenol®

15 - Generic name for Prevacid®

16 - Generic name for Remeron®

Common Drugs to be Avoided After Gastric Bypass

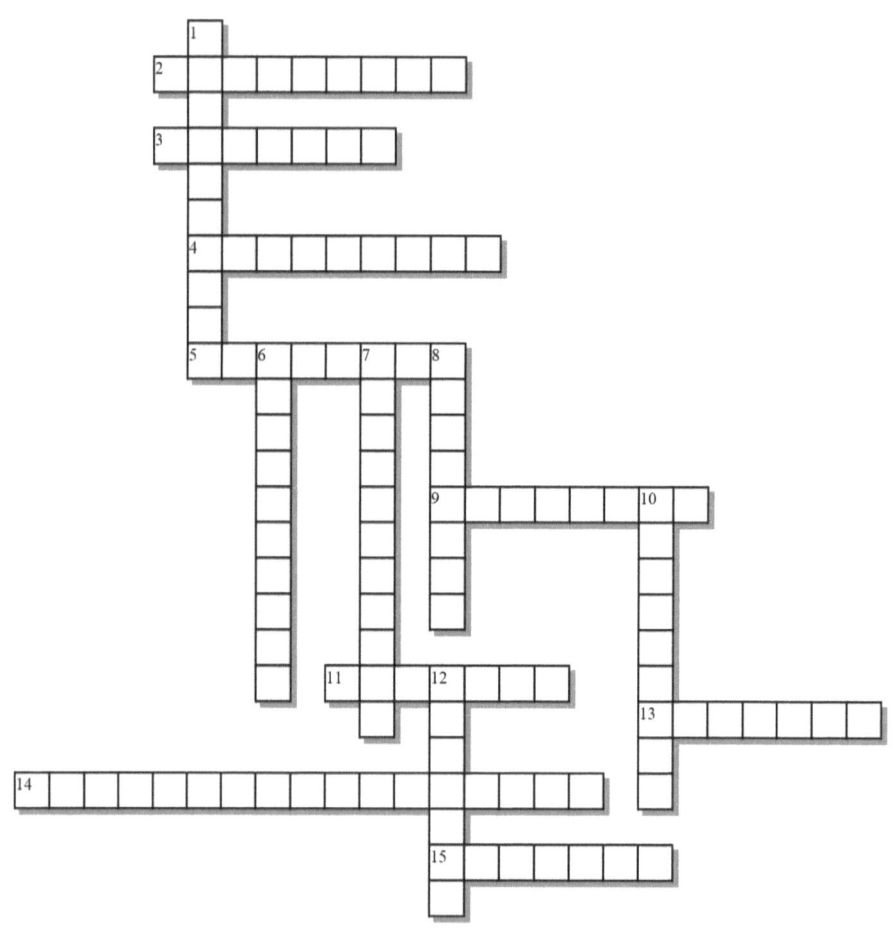

Across:

2 - Generic name for Celebrex®

3 - Brand name for diflunisal

4 - Generic name for Daypro®

5 - Brand name for naproxen

9 - Generic name for Tolectin®

11 - Brand name for alendronate

13 - Generic name for Piroxicam®

14 - Generic name for K-Dur®

15 - Another name for enteric-coated aspirin

Down:

1 - Generic name for Orudis®

6 - Generic name for Deltasone®

7 - Generic name for Methylprednisolone®

8 - Generic name for Habitrol®

10 - Generic name for Motrin®

12 - Brand name for risedronate

Common Drugs
Used in Blood Transfusion

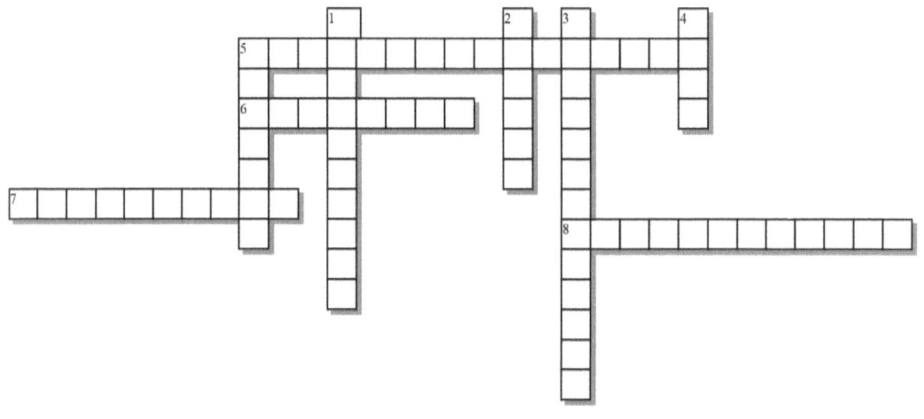

Across:

5 - Another term for a reaction that may present as indicated type I hypersensitivity response

6 - Another name for diphenhydramine, used as premedication prior to transfusion

7 - Lab value of blood (note: the other component of H/H)

8 - Only IV fluid used during blood transfusion to clear the line after infusions

Down:

1 - Lab value of blood (note: one of the H/H)

2 - Another name for hetastarch

3 Another name for Tylenol®, used as premedication prior to blood transfusion

4 - Measurement of blood

5 - Another name for human serum albumin

Common Drugs Used
in Palliative Care
for Comfort Measure

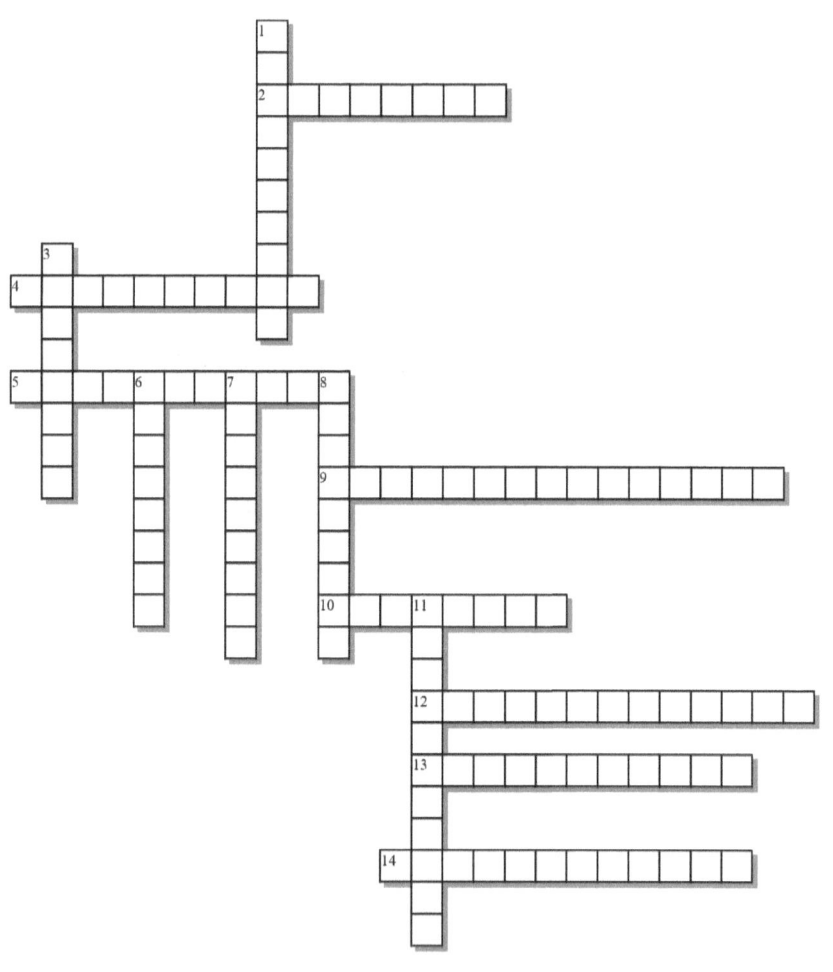

Across:

2 - Generic name for MS Contin®

4 - Generic name for Demerol®

5 - Generic name for Haldol®, used for agitation

9 - Lubricant eyedrops used for dry eyes

10 - Eyedrops that start with *A*, in the cholinergic category, this ophthalmic drop is used for promoting secretion

12 - Generic name for Tylenol®, used for pain

13 - Generic name for Transderm-Scop®

14. Generic name for Phenergan®, used for nausea

Down:

1 - Generic name for Pepcid®, for indigestion

3 - Generic name for Duragesic® or Sublimaze®

6 - Brand name for combo oxycodone/APAP, for pain

7 - Generic name for Motrin®

8 - Generic name for Ativan®, used for anxiety

11 - Generic name for Zofran®, used for nausea and vomiting

Common Drugs with
Black Box Warnings

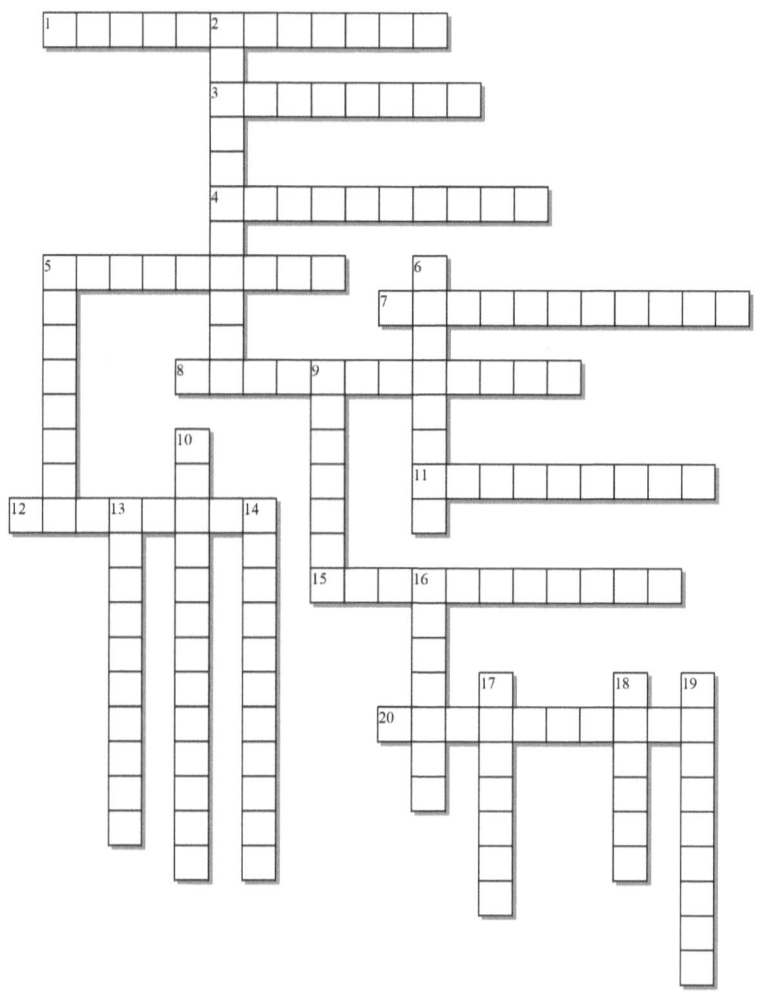

Across:

1 - Generic name for AmBisome® or Abelcet®

3 - Brand name for isotretinoin

4 - Generic name for Inapsine®

5 - Generic name for Felbatol®

7 - Generic name for Arava®

8 - Generic name for Nizoral®

11 - Generic name for Retin-A®

12 - Brand name for clozapine

15 - Generic name for Sandimmune®

20 - Generic name for Videx®

Down:

2 - Generic name for Thalomid®

5 - Generic name for Duragesic®

6 - Brand name for valproic acid

9 - Brand name for misoprostol

10 - Generic name for Tegretol®

13 - Generic name for Retrovir®

14 - Generic name for Lamictal®

16 - Generic name for Lithobid®

17 - Generic name for Danocrine®

18 - Brand name for ticlopidine

19 - Generic name for Toradol®

Common Heartburn Medications

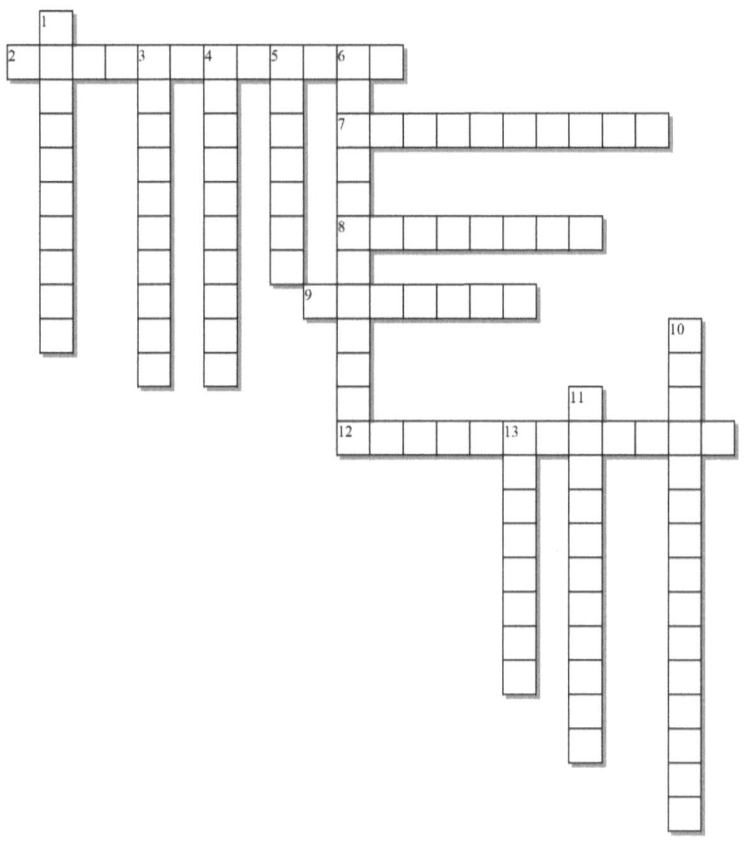

Across:

2 - Generic name for Protonix®

7 - Generic name for Axid®

8 - This brand-name drug is available as granules for patients who have nasogastric tubes

9 - Brand name for cimetidine

12 - Generic name for Nexium®

Down:

1 - Generic name for Pepcid®

3 - Generic name for Prilosec®

4 - Generic name for Zantac®

5 - A rapid-release form of omeprazole and sodium bicarbonate

6 - Generic name for Prevacid®

10 - Generic name for Dexilant®

11 - Generic name for Aciphex®

13 - This brand-name drug is available as a SoluTab

Common Medications
Cannot Be Crushed

```
E Y M K V K R S N I C A H T E M O D N I P Y
W A D D E R A L L X R N X O N E R G G A R P
S O F E N T A N Y L A C C O L A T E E N O C
U X O P A U G M E N T I N E X I U M Q I C I
D C S A M B I E N C R R F F V M G K C F A P
E A A K E C E T O R H T R A B D J G O E R R
X R M O N K A V O D A R T V I U F H N D D O
I D A T D I T R O P A N X L A R W Z C I I X
L I X E A D A L A T R X R O X E F F E P A R
A Z U L F I D I N E C O T R I N C C R I X P
N E N T O C O R T Q F C L M N D K U T N L J
T M U T S J P M U C I N E X X I T K A E R E
I J V F N A I D A K S K Y S L U P A W I U R
V N I A S P A N O Y C Y X C I T R O F Y M E
```

Accolate	Adalat	Adderall XR
Aggrenox	Ambien CR	Arthrotec
Augmentin	Avodart	Azulfidine
Biaxin XL	Cardizem	Cipro XR
Concerta	Depakote	Dexilant
Ditropan XL	Ecotrin	Effexor XR
Entocort	Fentanyl	Fosamax
Imdur	Indomethacin SR	Kadian
Mucinex	Myfortic	Namenda
Nexium	Niaspan	Nifedipine
Procardia XL	Toprol XL	

Common Medications
Used in Dialysis

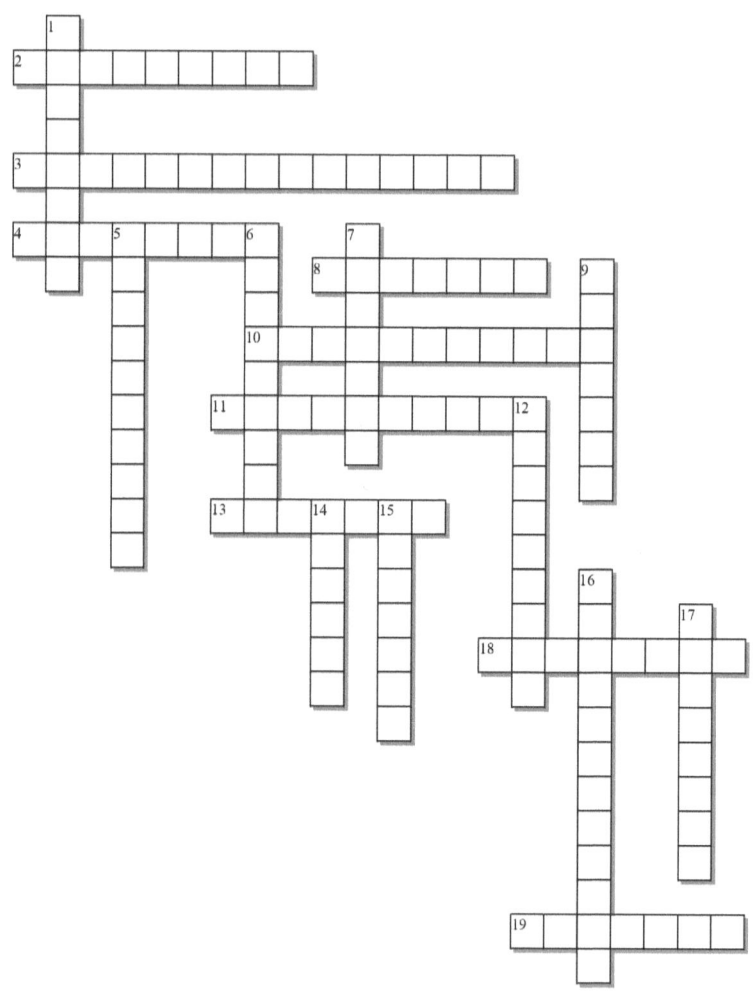

Across:

2 - Trade name for ferric gluconate, an intravenous iron

3 - Generic name for Benadryl®, used for itching/hives

4 - Generic name for Osmitrol®, used as an osmotic diuretic agent and a weak renal vasodilator

8 - Brand name for sevelamer

10 - Generic name for Zofran®, used for nausea and vomiting

11 - Generic name for Calcijex®, used to treat low calcium levels in the blood of patients undergoing chronic kidney dialysis

13 - Trade name for paricalcitol, used to treat secondary hyperparathyroidism in patients with chronic kidney failure

18 - Trade name for lanthanum carbonate

19 - Brand name for iron sucrose injection

Down:

1 - Trade name for cinacalcet, a calcimimetic, very effective in lowering PTH levels

5 - Trade name for vitamin B complex with C and folic acid

6 - Generic name for Xylocaine®, used as an anesthetic

7 - An IV blood thinner that starts with letter *H*

9 - Brand name for sevelamer carbonate

12 - Generic name for Trandate®, used for high blood pressure

14 - Brand name for calcium acetate

15 - Generic name for Albuminar®, used for hypotension in hemodialysis

16 - The most common IV fluid used in hemodialysis

17 - Generic name for MS Contin®, used for severe pain

Common Ophthalmic Medications

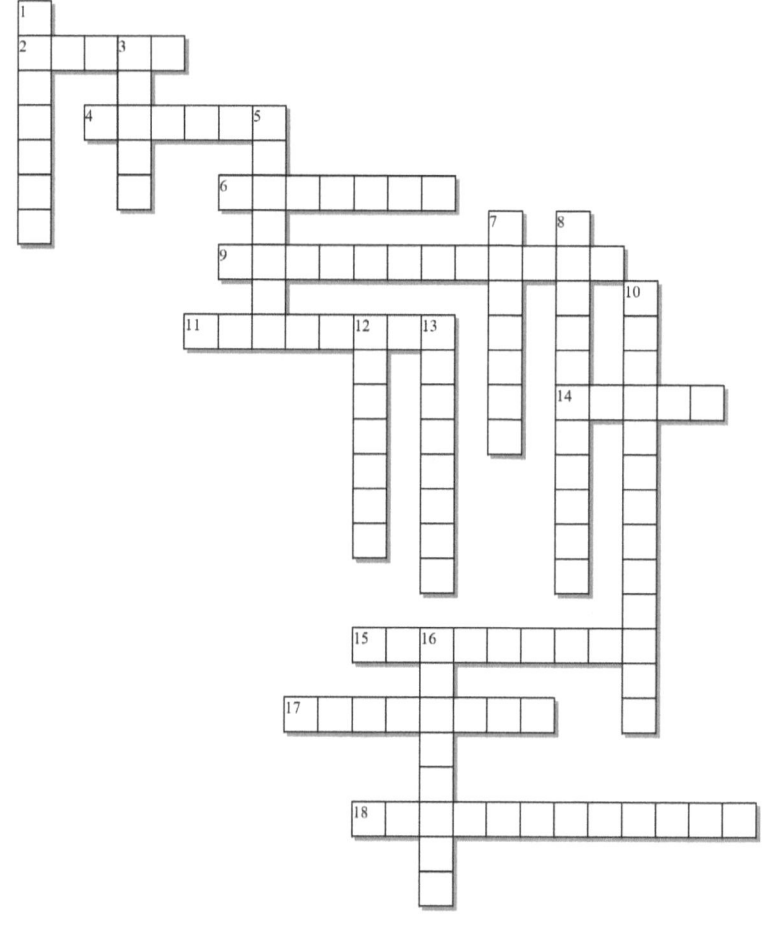

Across:

2 - Brand name for gatifloxacin, an ophthalmic antibiotic

4 - Brand name for the combination of dorzolamide and timolol, used for glaucoma

6 - Generic name for Bimatoprost®

9 - Generic name for Vigamox®, an antibiotic

11 - Brand name for betaxolol, used for glaucoma

14 - Brand name for loteprednol, anti-inflammatory eyedrops used to relieve seasonal allergies

15 - Generic name for Acular®, used for inflammation or swelling

17 - Brand name for brimonidine, used for glaucoma

18 - Generic name for Metipranolol®, beta-blocker eyedrops

Down:

1 - Brand name for azithromycin, used for the treatment of bacterial conjunctivitis

3 - Brand name for brinzolamide, a carbonic anhydrase inhibitor

5 - Brand name for dorzolamide

7 - Brand name for latanoprost

8 - Generic name for Pilopine®, a cholinergic medication used for promoting drainage of ocular fluids

10 - Generic name for Ciloxan®, an ophthalmic antibiotic

12 - Generic name for Timoptic®, a beta-blocker used for glaucoma

13 - Brand name for the combination of brimonidine and timolol, used for glaucoma

16 - Brand name for travoprost, a prostaglandin ophthalmic drop used to treat glaucoma

Common Pharmacy References

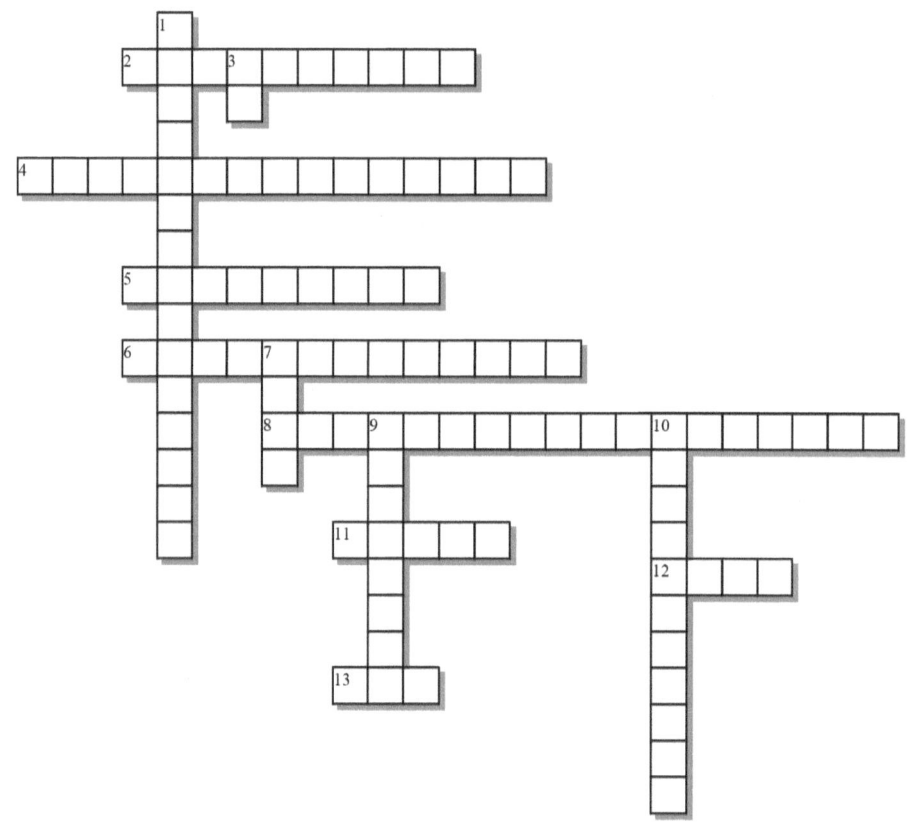

Across:

2 - This reference contains multisource drug products (generic drugs) that are bioequivalent

4 - This reference provides comprehensive information of drug-drug interaction

5 - This reference provides comprehensive drug information in pediatrics

6 - A complete labeling and dispensing information that goes with all drugs from the manufacturer

8 - This reference contains facts about all current medications in the United States and is updated monthly

11 - This reference contains an easy, lay-term-language type of information about drugs for patients to understand, is the abbreviation of *United States Pharmacopeia Dispensing Information*

12 - This reference is usually located in the intranet of each institution's settings and stands for *Material Safety and Data Sheet*

13 - This reference is the abbreviation of *United States Pharmacopeia*

Down:

1 - This reference provides comprehensive information of drug-drug interaction

3 - This reference is the abbreviation of *National Formulary*

7 - This reference is the abbreviation of *American Hospital Formulary Service*

9 - This reference was named after this man who came up with the most comprehensive source of injectable-drug information, such as compatibility and stability of most common drugs used in the hospitals

10 - This reference provides information about the laws and rules governing the practice of pharmacy in the state

Cytochrome P450
Enzyme Inducers

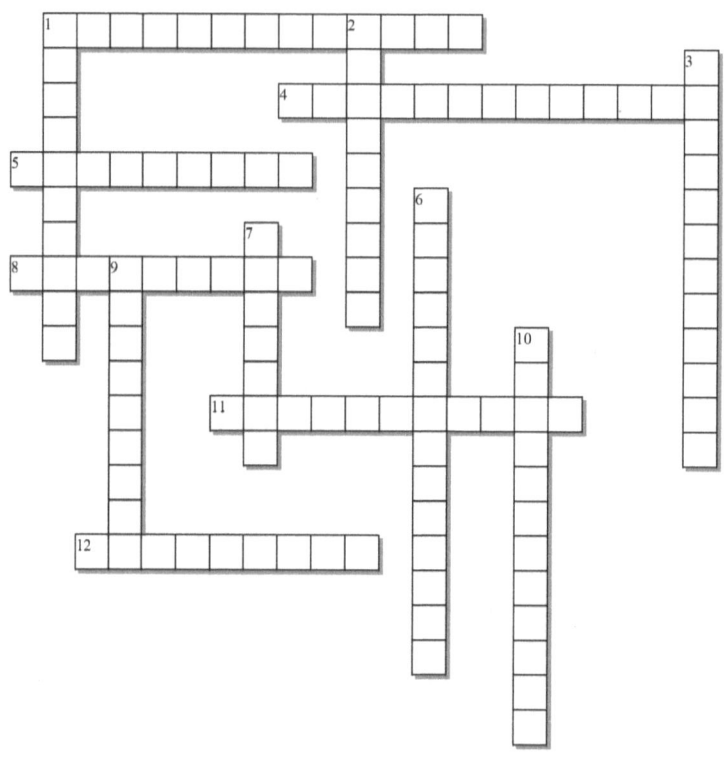

Across

1 - Generic name for Tegretol®, used for seizure

4 - Generic name for Luminal®, used for epilepsy

5 - Generic name for Mysoline®

8 - Generic name for Mycobutin®

11 - Generic name for Zocor®

12 - Generic name for Felbatol®

Down:

1 - Generic name for Zyrtec®

2 - Generic name for Dilantin®, antiseizure drug

3 - Generic name for Lotrimin®, an antifungal

6 - Generic name for Questran®

7 - Trade name for rifampin

9 - Brand name for spironolactone

10 - Generic name for Gris-PEG®

Cytochrome P450 Enzyme Inhibitors

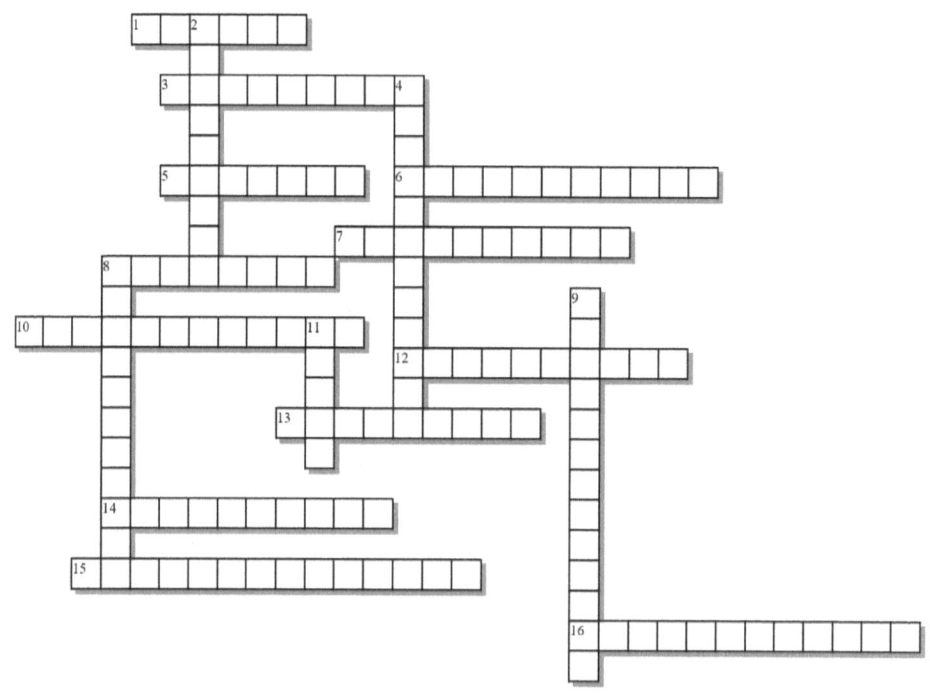

Across:

1 - Brand name for fenofibrate

3 - Brand name for amiodarone, an antiarrhythmic

5 - Trade name for nicardipine

6 - Generic name for Ticlid®, used for circulation

7 - Generic name for Zoloft®

8 - Brand name for diltiazem, used for blood pressure

10 - Generic name for Nizoral®, an antifungal

12 - Generic name for Celexa®, used for depression

13 - Generic name for Norvir®, an antiviral

14 - Generic name for Ranexa®, a heart med

15 - Generic name for Biaxin®, an antibiotic

16 - Generic name for Sporanox®

Down:

2 - Generic name for Nydrazid®

4 - Generic name for Eryc®, an antibiotic

8 - Generic name for Plavix®

9 - Generic name for Cipro®, an antibiotic

11 - Brand name for gemfibrozil

Diabetic Medications
and Supplies

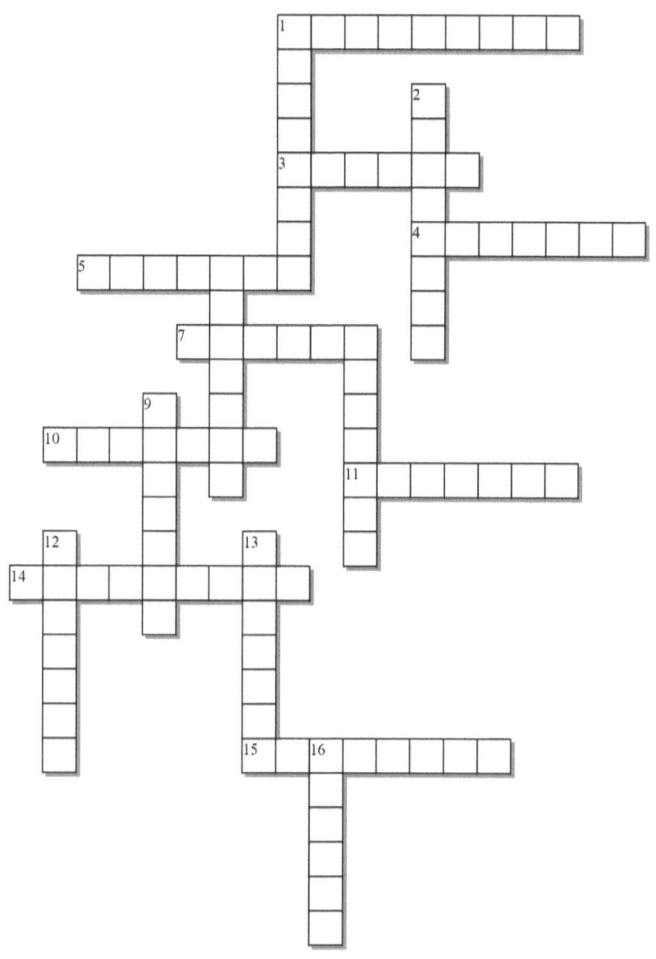

Across:

1 - Generic name for Glucotrol®

3 - Brand name for glulisine

4 - Brand name for aspart

5 - Brand name for repaglinide

7 - Brand name for glargine

10 - Brand name for sitagliptin

11 - This device is used in conjunction with the glucometer to give the reading of the patient's blood sugar

14 - Generic name for Glucophage®

15 - Generic name for Precose®

Down:

1 - Medication used in the treatment of hypoglycemia

2 - Used to give insulin subcutaneously

6 - Test strip used in treating diabetes

8 - Brand name for nateglinide

9 - Brand name for lispro

12 - Brand name for detemir

13 - Brand name for glyburide

16 - Brand name for glimepiride

Different Practice Sites

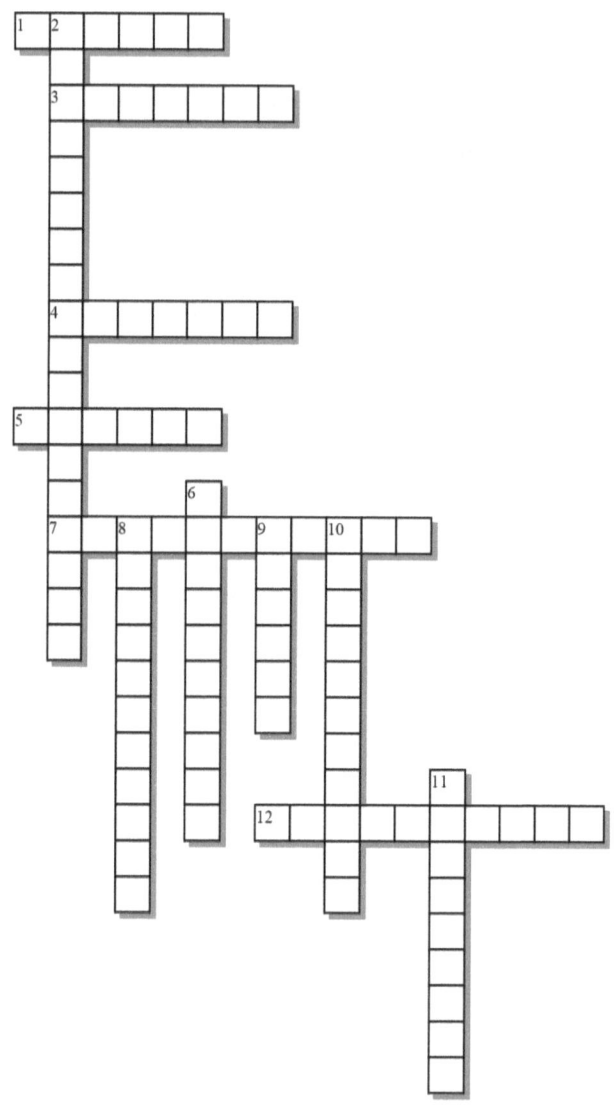

Across:

1 - This class is where ambulatory care or community pharmacies are classified

3 - This site is class B pharmacy only

4 - This site is where palliative care is provided for comfort care during the end stage of cancer

5 - This site is class D pharmacy, supervised by a physician

7 - This site specializes in hormone and other nonsterile compounding products

12 - This site is class E, mails out prescriptions to patients

Down:

2 - This site is where older patients with chronic illness transfer to and it provides a range of services and supports to the patient over a long period of time

6 - This site is where patients obtain their IV medications after being discharged from the hospital

8 - Where health insurance companies are managed

9 - Maximum number of days patients receive from mail order

10 - Another name for hospital pharmacy

11 - Another name for retail pharmacy

Different Routes of Administration

```
E C P V H C N O I T A L A H N I Y G U V Y C
S D O B M L M M J T C P U I P G P G S T M S
U L A P V I - S C I H I O I G M I - N O O U
O A J E Y E D R O P N I R R H - T J Y A T O
N M I P R G I B U I R T L T D D T N O C S E
E R L N P O R A L J B O R A S R D L J Y O N
V E R A J U S U J Y S P V A T A A H U D R A
A D A S I E B O J C G I S A T C G E V Y T T
R A G A S B C G L Y M C E D G H E O J J S U
T R A L U C I T R A - A R T N I E R S G A C
N T T L O L C P I M I L M C T L N C E A G B
I N M Y L V C U S O H Y M T R N U A A M N U
D I H B U S Y T R A N S D E R M A L L L C S
D U T R A L U C S U M A R T N I - D G C R -
```

Aerosol	Ear drop	Eye drop
Gastrostomy	Inhalation	Injection
Intra-articular	Intradermal	Intramuscular
Intrathecal	Intravenous	Nasally
Nasogastric	Oral	Rectal
Subcutaneous	Topical	Transdermal
Vaginal		

Different Types of
Dosage Forms

```
Z C B Q A T A Z T C R E A M S T I Y R N S C
W V B F P M U L T I P L E D O S E F A P S S
L Q T F L A I X W R V A K K Z H J K X A U C
K T V Q V K K E S E S O D E L G N I S T P O
C L S M T I N C U T N B U L X W U Q S C P L
A A D E T A O C B N O I N T M E N T C H O L
B M P O W D E R L E I N J E C T I B L E S O
Y U P S O L U T I O N H P A D Y B B J W I D
G C C U U S Q A N A V A C C I N E S S A T I
G R J C L L P H G T E L B A T H E Y E B O O
I E T Y A E E R U Q B E L I X I R H O L R N
P A S T E L F E A X T R I O A U G W P E Y E
T M A D D S O P L Y G S U S P E N S I O N M
M A F P R B F U E F F E R V E S C E N T I Z
```

Ampule	Buccal	capsule
Chewable	Coated	Collodion
Cream	effervescent	Elixir
Enteric	inhaler	Injectible
Multiple dose	Ointment	Paste
Patch	Piggy back	Powder
Single dose	Solution	Spray
Sublingual	Suppository	Suspension
Syrup	Tablet	Vaccines

Different Types of Vaccines

```
X L U F L V R U B E L L A S S V Y E I H X L
J A B H L F L Y P L Q H I U F R U U R I V A
A C K E A D N R M M D N B J H Y M Q E Z P C
S C X P G D L F K I F R D B E P J A T O X C
T O H A I G T N O L A X S L S R Y L S K O O
I C I T B Y N H U B O U L U U S F P O R P C
T O J I C L P E I P L O R A K J F X Z P N O
A N H T T Y N E L I W I S E L S A E M A E M
P I W I T Z S L H F V S C H O L E R A D K U
E G L S A M A P E O L E V K G I T T V T C E
H N F B U M O V I H C A S U N A T E T S I N
W E O D S M E L T C J G R I I D D H M B H P
Z M M Z E R O V A R I C E L L A K O Z F C X
I M W H T P I X A V A T S O Z X A O Y B Y G
```

Chickenpox	Cholera	Hemophilus B
Hepatitis B	Hepatits A	Influenza
Measles	Menginococcal	MMR
Plaque	Pneumococcal	Poliovirus
Rabies	Rubella	Smallpox
Tdap	Tetanus	Typhoid
Varicella	Yellow Fever	Zostavax
Zoster		

Drugs that Commonly Interact with Grapefruit Juice

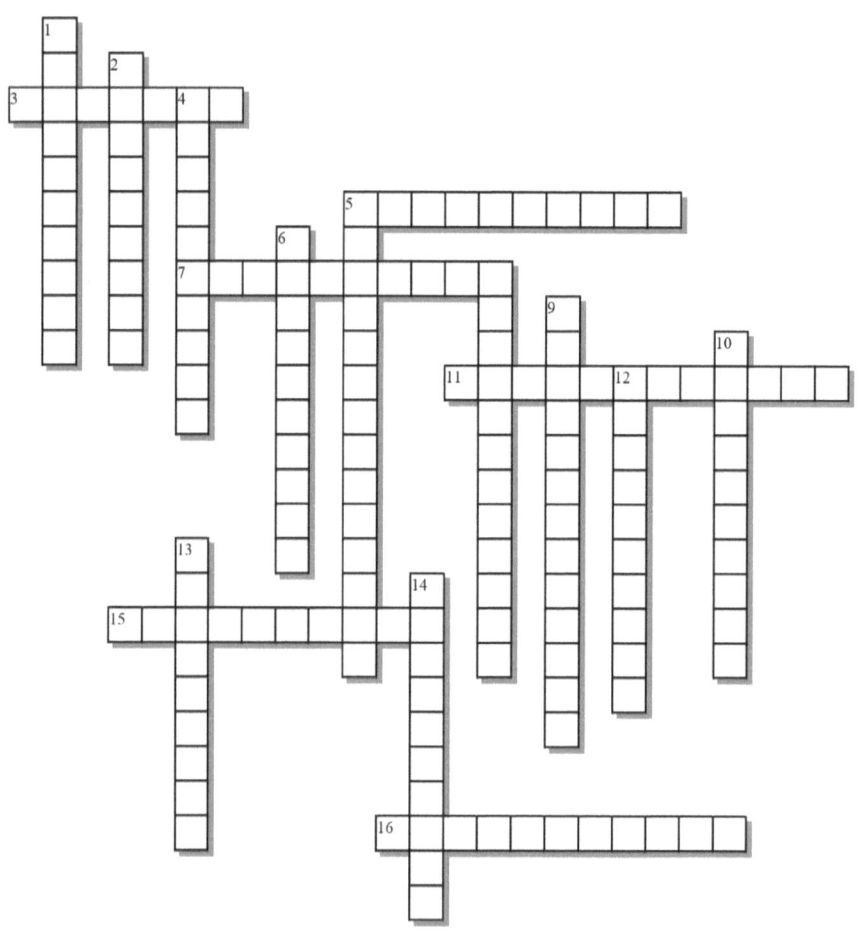

Across:

3 - Brand name for fexofenadine

5 - Generic for Colcrys®

7 - Generic for Cordarone®, can interact with grapefruit juice

11 - Generic for Lipitor®, can interact with grapefruit juice

15 - Generic for Claritin®

16 - Generic for Zocor®

Down:

1 - Generic for Viagra®

2 - Generic for Calan®

4 - Generic for Ranexa®

5 - Generic for Biaxin®

6 - Generic for Mevacor®

8 - Generic for Ery-Tab®

9 - Generic for Tegretol®

10 - Generic for Levitra®

12 - Generic for Xanax®, can have serious interaction with grapefruit juice

13 - Brand name for fentanyl

14 - Generic for Plendil®, can interact with grapefruit juice

Ear Drop Medications

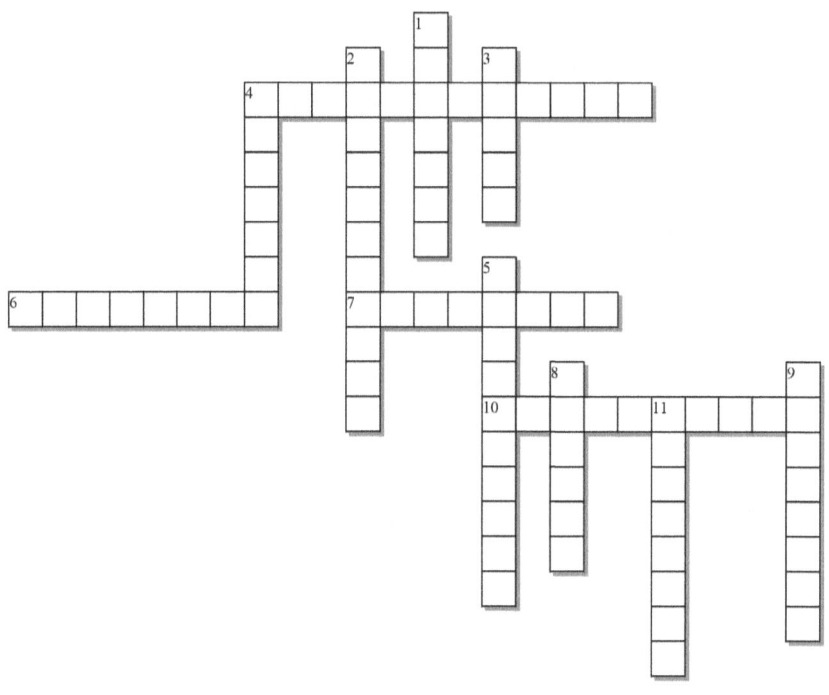

Across:

4 - Generic name for DermOtic® Oil ear drop, a steroid ear drop

6 - Brand name for this combo ear drop, antipyrine and benzocaine, an anesthetic ear drop used to reduce ear pain

7 - This type of oil has a medicinal purpose for aiding in ear pain relief by heating the oil

10 - Trade name for benzocaine, an anesthetic drop

Down:

1 - Brand name for isopropyl alcohol

2 - Brand name for hydrocortisone/neomycin/polymyxin B

3 - Brand name for acetic acid

4 - Brand name for ofloxacin, an anti-infective ear drop

5 - Generic name for Garamycin®

8 - Brand name for carbamide peroxide, an earwax softener

9 - Another brand name for neomycin, polymyxin B, and hydrocortisone ear drop

11 - Trade name for ciprofloxacin/dexamethasone

Hormone Medications

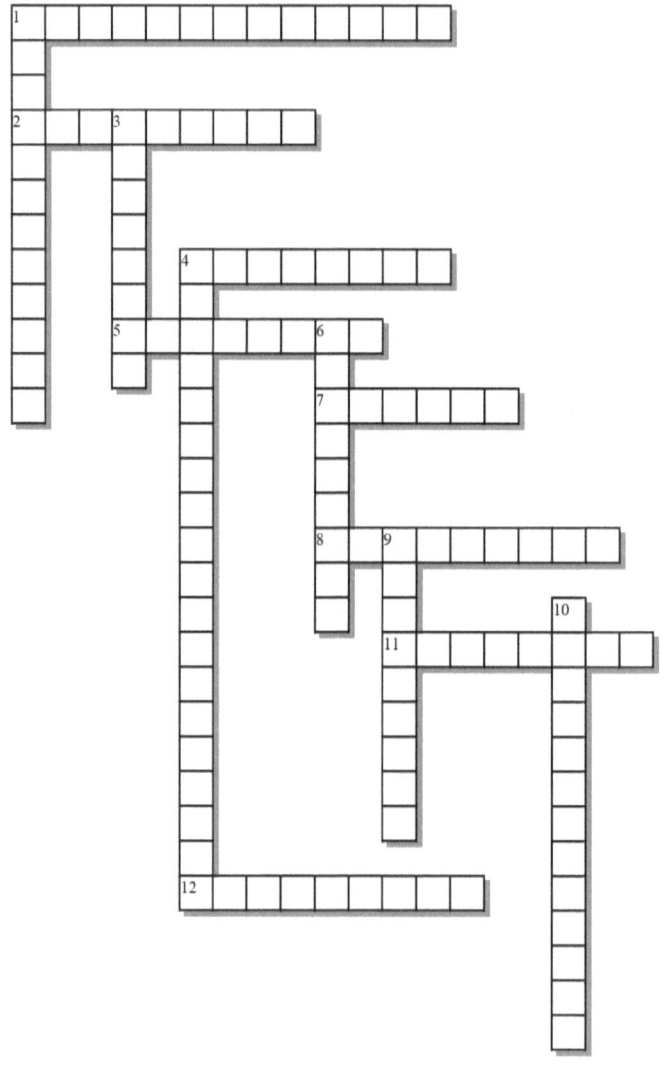

Across:

1 - Generic name for Synthroid®

2 - Brand name for testosterone patch

4 - Brand name for monophasic birth control pills

5 - Brand name for testosterone gel

7 - Brand name for testosterone capsule

8 - Generic name for Estrace®

11 - Another name for conjugated estrogen

12 - Brand name of esterified estrogen and testosterone

Down:

1 - Generic name for Cytomel®

3 - Brand name for Liotrix®

4 - Generic name for Provera®

6 - One of the brand names for estradiol patches

9 - Brand name for triphasic birth control pills

10 - Brand name for desiccated thyroid

Human Immunodeficiency Virus (HIV) Medications

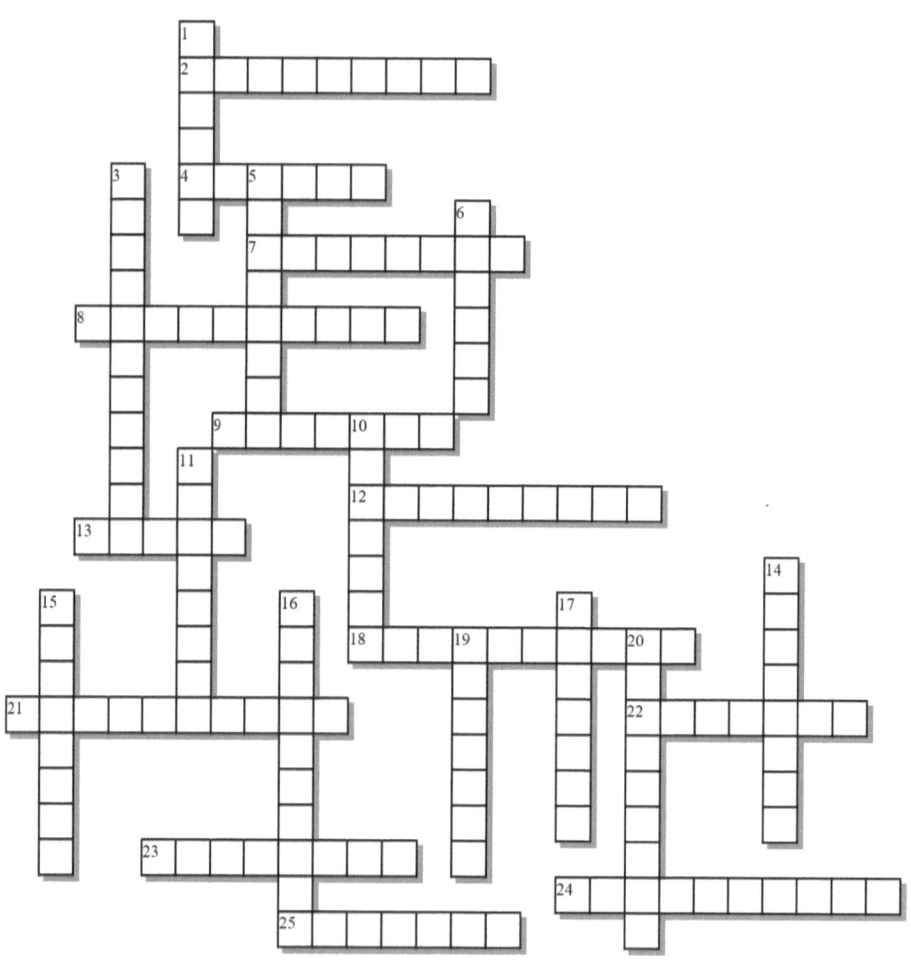

Across:

2 - Generic name for Sustiva®

4 - Brand name for tenofovir

7 - Brand name for combo (abacavir + lamivudine + zidovudine)

8 - Generic name for Videx®

9 - Trade name for combo (emtricitabine + tenofovir)

12 - Generic name for Norvir®

13 - Trade name for stavudine

18 - Generic name for Agenerase®

21 - Generic name for Invirase/Fortovase®

22 - Brand name for combo (abacavir + lamivudine)

23 - Trade name for combo (lamivudine + zidovudine)

24 - Brand name for delavirdine

Down:

1 - Trade name for fosamprenavir

3 - Generic name for Hivid®

5 - Brand name for zidovudine

6 - Brand name for abacavir

10 - Trade name for this combo med (emtricitabine + tenofovir + efavirenz)

11 - Brand name for indinavir

14 - Brand name for nelfinavir

15 - Trade name for nevirapine

16 - Generic name for Epivir®

17 - Trade name for this combo med (lopinavir + ritonavir)

19 - Brand name for stazanavir

20 - Trade name for raltegravir

25 - Trade name for emtricitabine

Intravenous Medications
that Require In-LineFilters

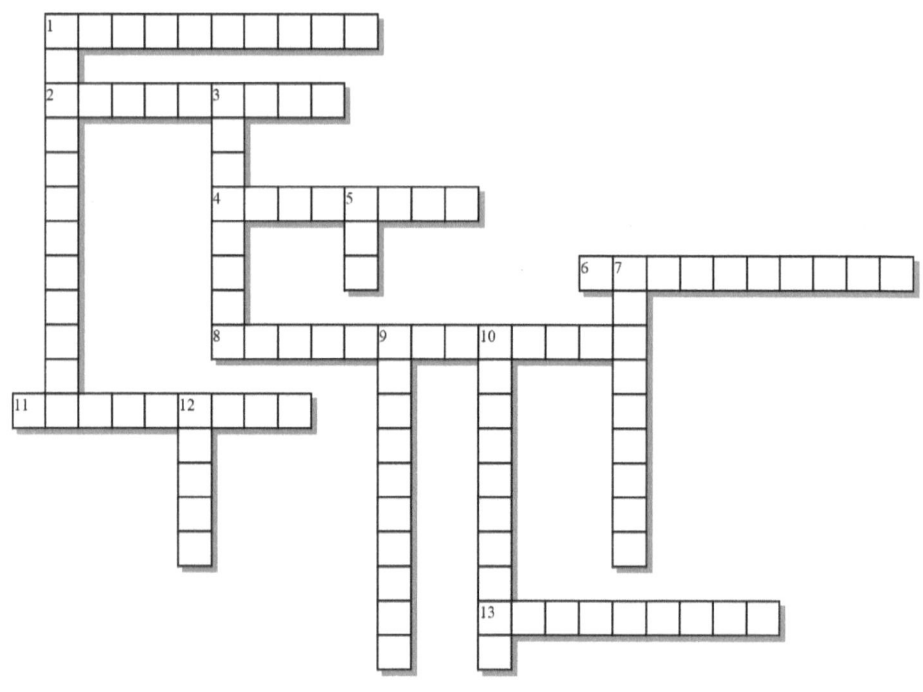

Across:

1 - Generic name for Cordarone®

2 - Generic name for Dilantin®, used for seizures

4 - Brand name for mannitol

6 - Generic name for this cytotoxic drug Taxol®

8 - Generic name for AmBisome®, an antifungal injection

11 - Generic name for Retavase®, a thrombolytic drug

13 - Generic name for Reopro®, a platelet aggregation inhibitor

Down:

1 - Generic name for Elspar®, an anticancer drug

3 - Generic name for Thioplex®, an anticancer drug

5 - The abbreviation for total parenteral nutrition

7 - Brand name for albumin

9 - Generic name for this cytotoxic drug Vumon®

10 - Generic name for Remicade®, a monoclonal antibody against tumor

12 - Another name for fatty emulsion

Non-steroidal Anti-inflammatory Medications

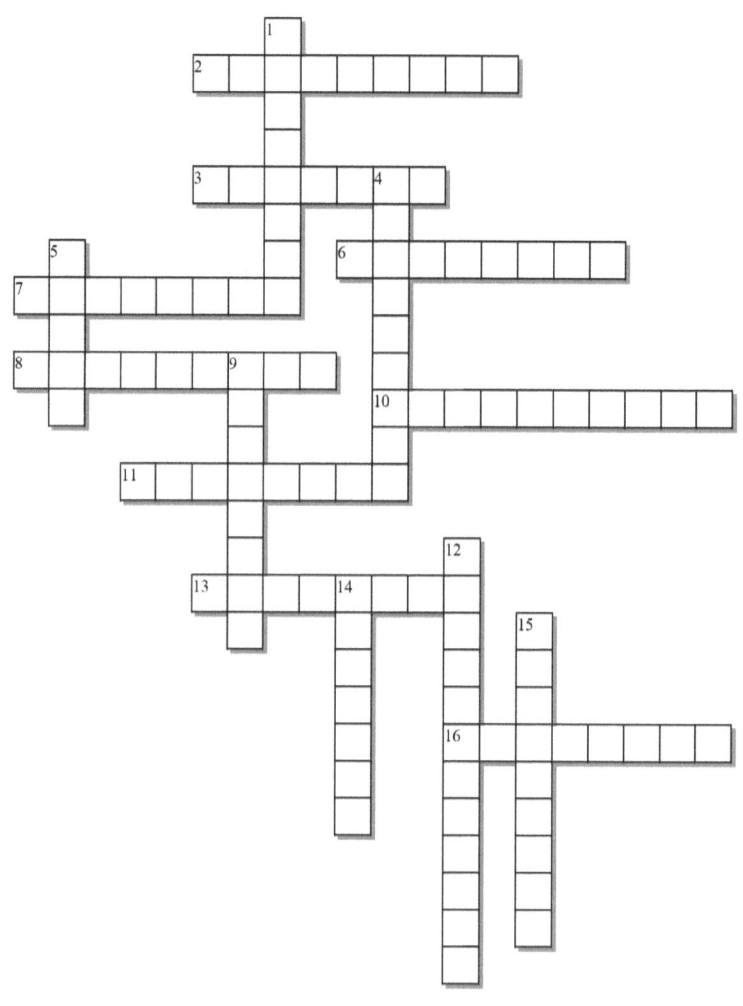

Across:

2 - Generic name for Daypro®

3 - This brand-name aspirin is available as an enteric-coated tablet

6 - Generic name for Clinoril®

7 - Trade name for diclofenac

8 - Generic name for Feldene®

10 - Generic name for Nalfon®

11 - Trade name for tolmetin

13 - Trade name for meclofenamate

16 - Generic name for Lodine®

Down:

1 - Trade name for naproxen

4 - Generic name for Motrin®

5 - Brand name for meloxicam

9 - Trade name for celecoxib

12 - Generic name for Indocin®

14 - Brand name for ketoprofen

15 - Generic name for Toradol®, and it is used widely in most institutional settings

Osteoporosis Medications

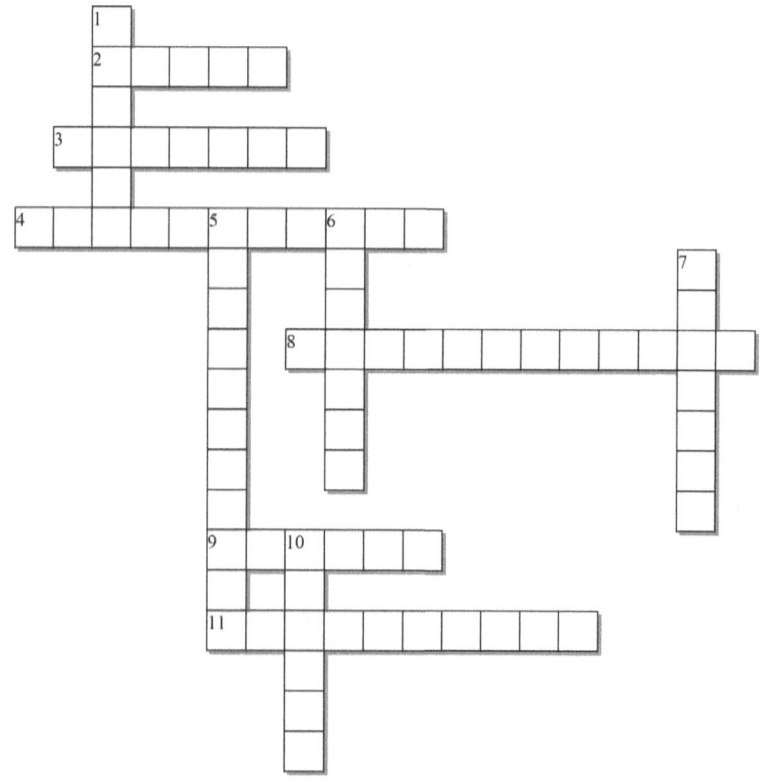

Across:

2 - An OTC brand of calcium

3 - Brand name for zoledronic acid

4 - Generic name for Boniva®

8 - This brand-name drug is a combo of alendronate/ cholecalciferol

9 - Trade name for pamidronate

11 - Generic name for Didronel®

Down:

1 - Brand name for zoledronic acid

5 - Generic name for Actonel®

6 - This brand-name medication is also available with calcium, starts with letter *A*

7 - Trade name for alendronate

10 - Trade name for raloxifene

Over-the-Counter
Medications

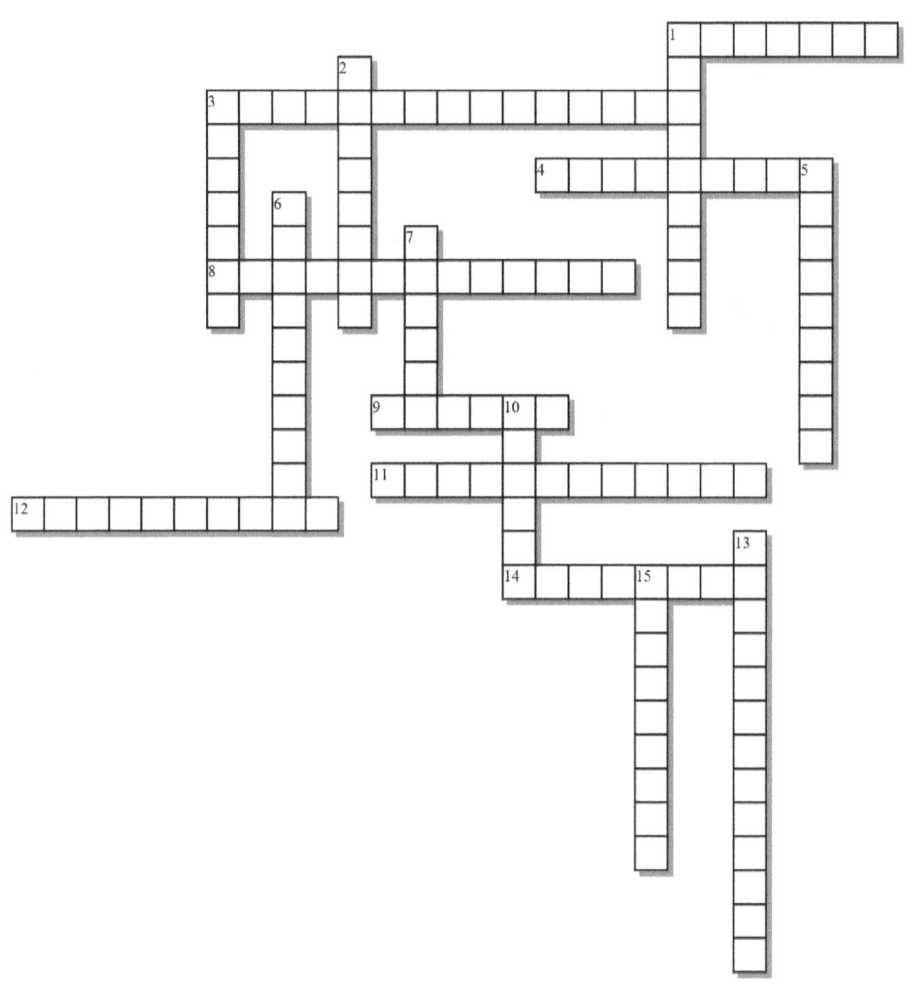

Across:

1 - Another name for common vitamin found over-the-counter

3 - Generic name for this medication which is used in treating hives, itching, or allergic reactions

4 - Generic name for Motrin®, used in mild pain or other inflammation relief

8 - Generic name for Tylenol®, used for headache, pain, or fever

9 - Name this ear drop that is used in removal of earwax

11 - A brand of medication that is used in treating hemorrhoids

12 - Another name for saline nasal spray (OTC)

14 - Drug used in treating antifungal athlete's foot

Down:

1 - Name this cream that is used in daily clear acne treatment

2 - Another brand name for famotidine

3 - Another name for bisacodyl, which is available in both tablet and suppository forms

5 - Another name for a triple antibiotic used in treating minor cuts, scrapes, or abrasions

6 - Name this saline enema that is used in constipation

7 - Eyedrops used in treating relief redness of eyes

10 - This OTC brand-name med is used for severe toothache pain relief

13 - Type of test strip used in testing blood sugar (starts with "One")

15 - Another brand name for loperamide (OTC)

Pain Medications (Narcotic)

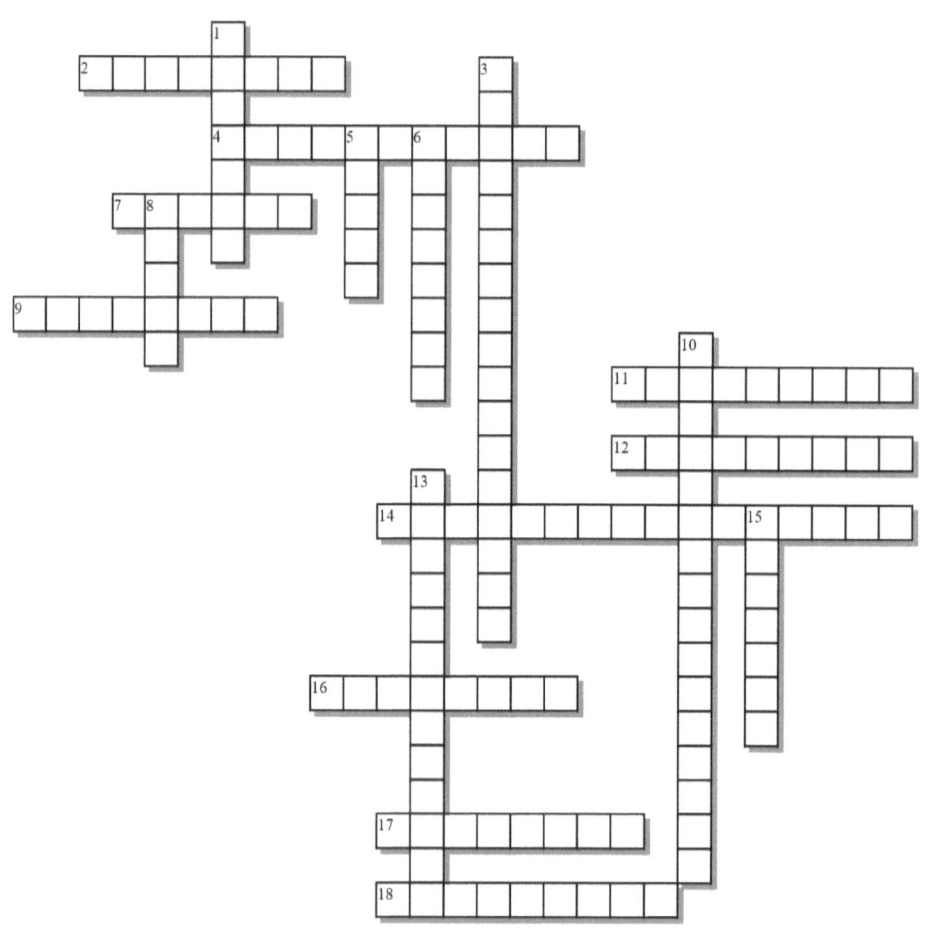

Across:

2 - Brand name for oxycodone/ aspirin

4 - Generic name for Opana®

7 - Brand name for morphine sustained-release capsule

9 - Trade name for pentazocine and naloxone

11 - Generic name for Oxycontin®

12 - Brand name for fentanyl

14 - Trade name for acetaminophen w/ codeine

16 - Brand name for buprenorphine and naloxone

17 - Generic name for MS Contin®

18 - Generic name for Dolophine®

Down:

1 - Trade name for diphenoxylate and atropine

3 - Trade name for butalbital, APAP, and caffeine w/ codeine

5 - Trade name for immediate-release oxycodone

6 - Brand name for oxycodone/ APAP

8 - Trade name for rapid-action fentanyl oral swab

10 - Generic name for Vicodin® or Lortab®

13 - Generic name for Dilaudid®

15 - Brand name for meperidine

Pain Medications (Nonnarcotic)

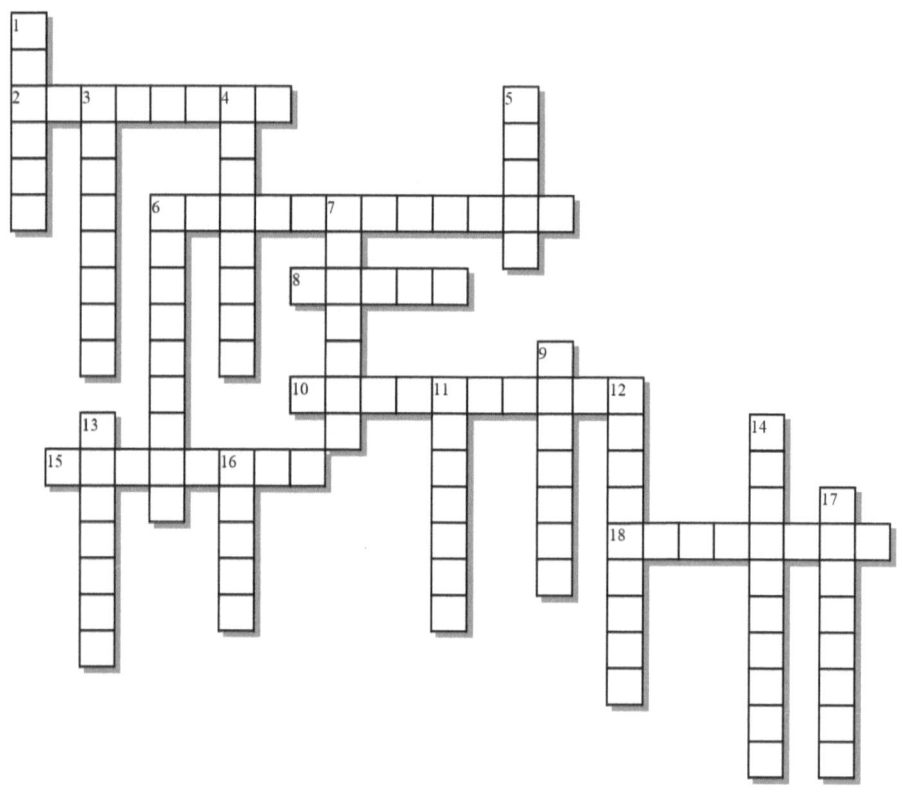

Across:

2 - Trade name for a combo of tramadol and acetaminophen

6 - Generic name for Indocin®

8 - Brand name for meloxicam

10 - Generic name for Voltaren®

15 - An OTC brand name for Tylenol® suppository

18 - Another trade name for ibuprofen injection

Down:

1 - An OTC brand name for ketoprofen

3 - Generic name for Ultram®

4 - Generic name for Lodine®

5 - The abbreviation for nonsteroidal anti-inflammatory drugs

6 - Generic name for Motrin®

7 - An enteric-coated form of aspirin

9 - Another trade name for naproxen

11 - A brand name for acetaminophen injection

12 - Generic name for Celebrex®

13 - Trade name for nabumetone

14 - Generic name for Oruvail®

16 - Brand name for naproxen

17 - Trade name for Tolmetin®

Penicillin and Cephalosporin Antibiotics

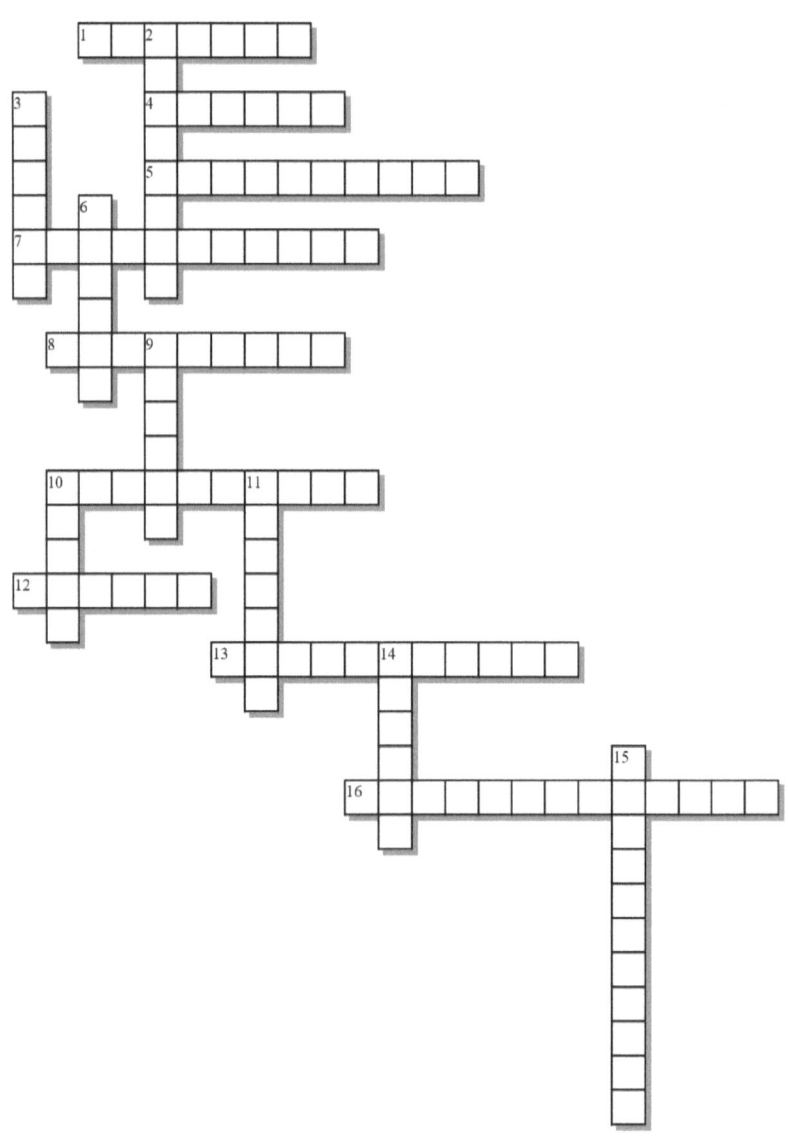

Across:

1 - Brand name for cefadroxil

4 - Brand name for cefaclor

5 - Generic name for Pen VK® or Veetids®

7 - Generic name for Amoxil®

8 - Another name for Nafcil®

10 - Generic name for Principen®

12 - Brand name for cephalexin

13 - Generic name for Ticar®

16 - Generic name for Zosyn®

Down:

2 - Brand name for ceftriaxone

3 - Brand name for cefixime

6 - Brand name for ceftazidime

9 - Brand name for cefuroxime

10 - Brand name for cefazolin

11 - Brand name for loracarbef

14 - Brand name for cefprozil

15 - Generic name for Tegopen®

Pharmacy
Health Insurance Review

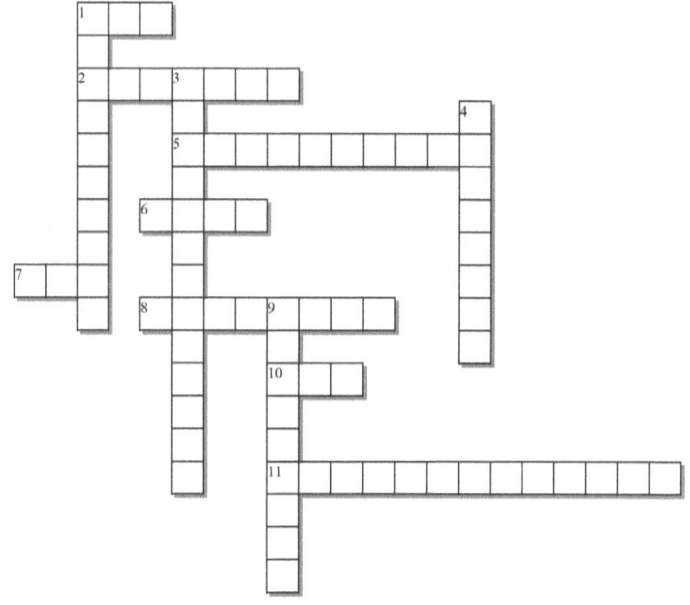

Across:

1 - The abbreviation for Central Medicare Services

2 - An amount set by the health insurance company paid monthly by the patient for coverage

5 - An amount the patient has to pay before their co-payment is applied

6 - The abbreviation for National Committee for Quality Assurance

7 - The abbreviation for Health Maintenance Organization

8 - A type of state insurance provided by the Department of Health and Human Services for low-income patients

10 - The abbreviation for Preferred Provider Organization

11 - A type of government insurance that pays for patients sixty-five years or older to cover their medications

Down:

1 - A fee paid by a patient to a provider for management of patient's health care even if the patient does not seek care

3 - A type of government insurance that pays for patients sixty-five years or older to cover their medical and hospital fees

4 - A type of federal insurance that covers for patients sixty-five years or older

9 - An amount set by the health insurance for services or medications provided for a patient

Pharmacy Technician Duties

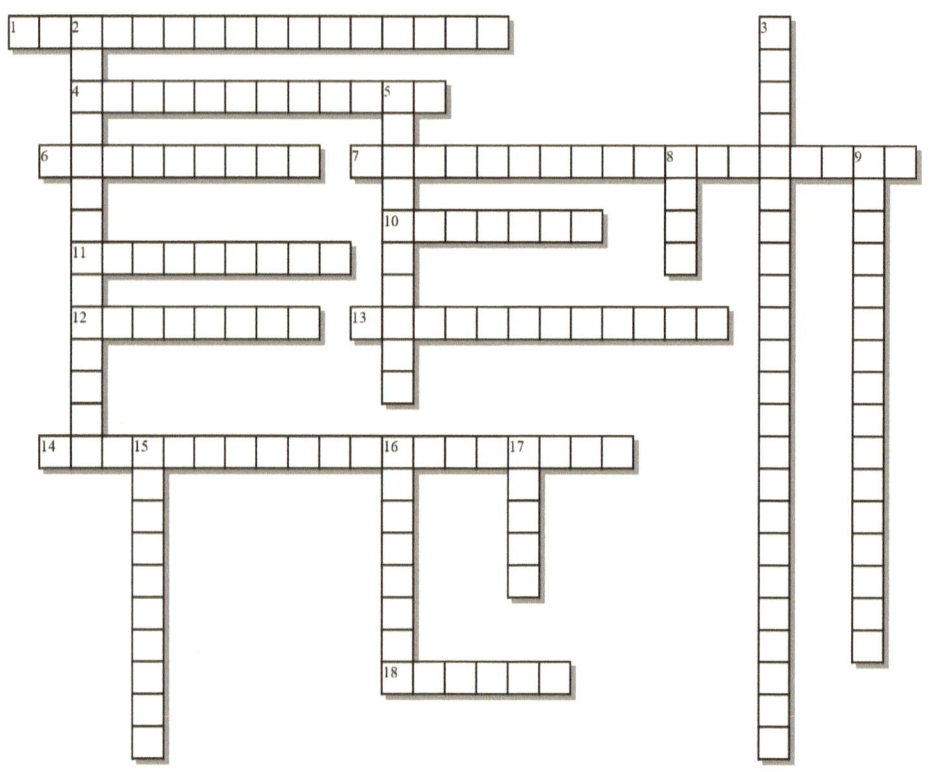

Across:

1 - A procedure that is performed under sterile condition with the goal of minimizing contamination

4 - An order written by a physician for the patient

6 - Another name for *trade name*

7 - Obtained from the patient prior to entering data into the system

10 - Another name for *nonproprietary name*

11 - A way to keep track of products on hand

12 - Another name for *controlled substances*

13 - A service where the pharmacist discusses to the patient about their medication prior to their taking the medication

14 - A title obtained after passing the national board tech exam

18 - Call physician's office to ask for more

Down:

2 - The length of the product is set by the manufacturer based on its stability

3 - Another name for drugs that are chemically different but have the same therapeutic outcome and similiar toxicities

5 - This book lists approved drug products with therapeutic equivalence evaluation

8 - The abbreviation of the Omnibus Budget Reconciliation Act

9 - A type of medication that does not need a prescription from a doctor

15 - Another name for the insurance

16 - Patient's pertinent data is entered into this machine

17 - An amount the patient has to pay after submitting through insurance

Respiratory Medications

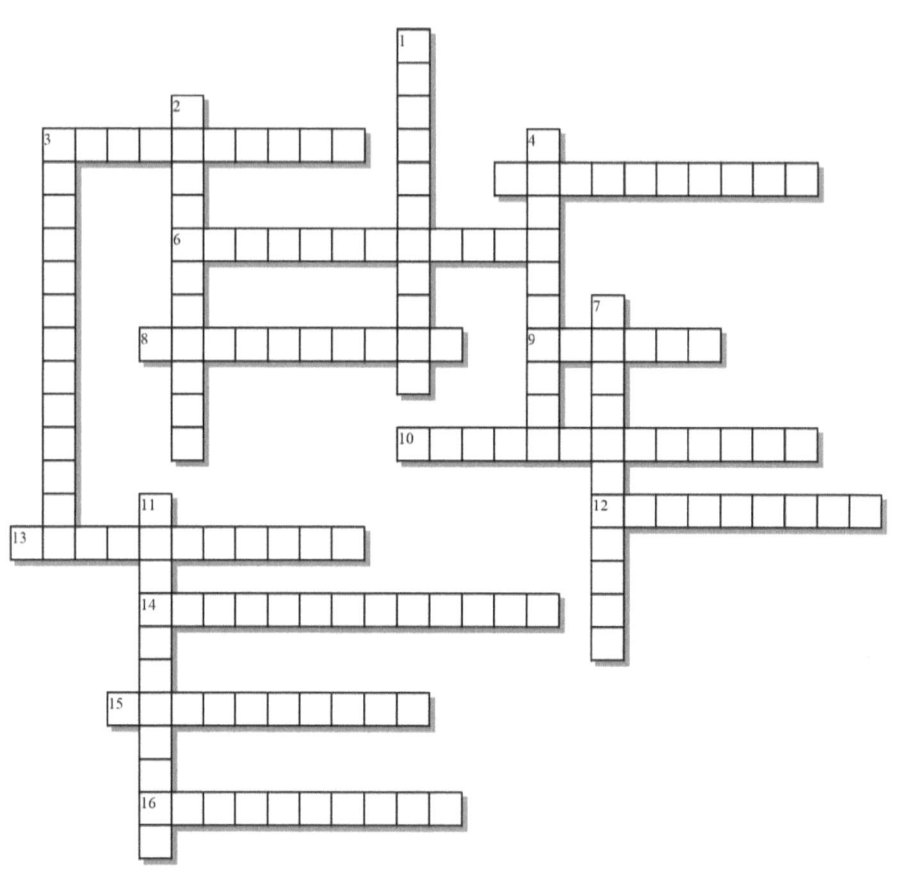

Across:

3 - Generic name for Maxair®

5 - Generic name for Claritin®

6 - Another name for Allegra®

8 - Generic name for Zyrtec®

9 - Main ingredient in Ocean nasal spray

10 - Generic name for Afrin®

12 - Generic name for Proventil HFA®

13 - Generic name for Tessalon® Perles

14 - Generic name for Azmacort®

15 - Generic name for Pulmicort®

16 - Generic name for Serevent® inhaler

Down:

1 - Generic name for Flonase®

2 - Main ingredient of Robitussin®

3 - Main ingredient of Neo-Synephrine®

4 - Generic name for Nasonex®

7 - Generic name for Patanol®

11 - Generic name for Singulair®

Topical Acne Medications

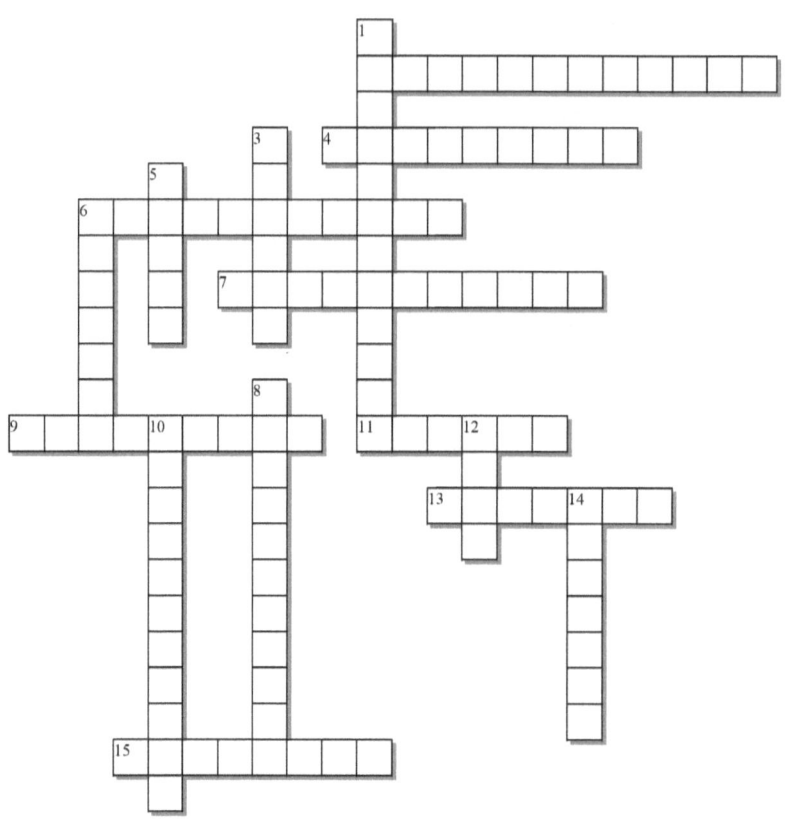

Across:

2 - Generic name for Erygel®

4 - Generic name for Retin-A Micro® gel

6 - Generic name for Evoclin®

7 - Generic name for Adoxa®

9 - Trade name for benzoyl peroxide and clindamycin

11 - Brand name for adapalene and benzoyl peroxide

13 - Trade name for tazarotene

15 - Brand name for adapalene

Down:

1 - Generic name for Sumycin®

3 - Trade name for sodium sulfacetamide, used as facial lotion

5 - Trade name for combo clindamycin and tretinoin

6 - Trade name for clindamycin gel

8 - Generic name for Minocin®

10 - Generic name for Finacea® or Azelex®

12 - Brand name for benzoyl peroxide and clindamycin

14 - Trade name for tretinoin

Topical Steroids

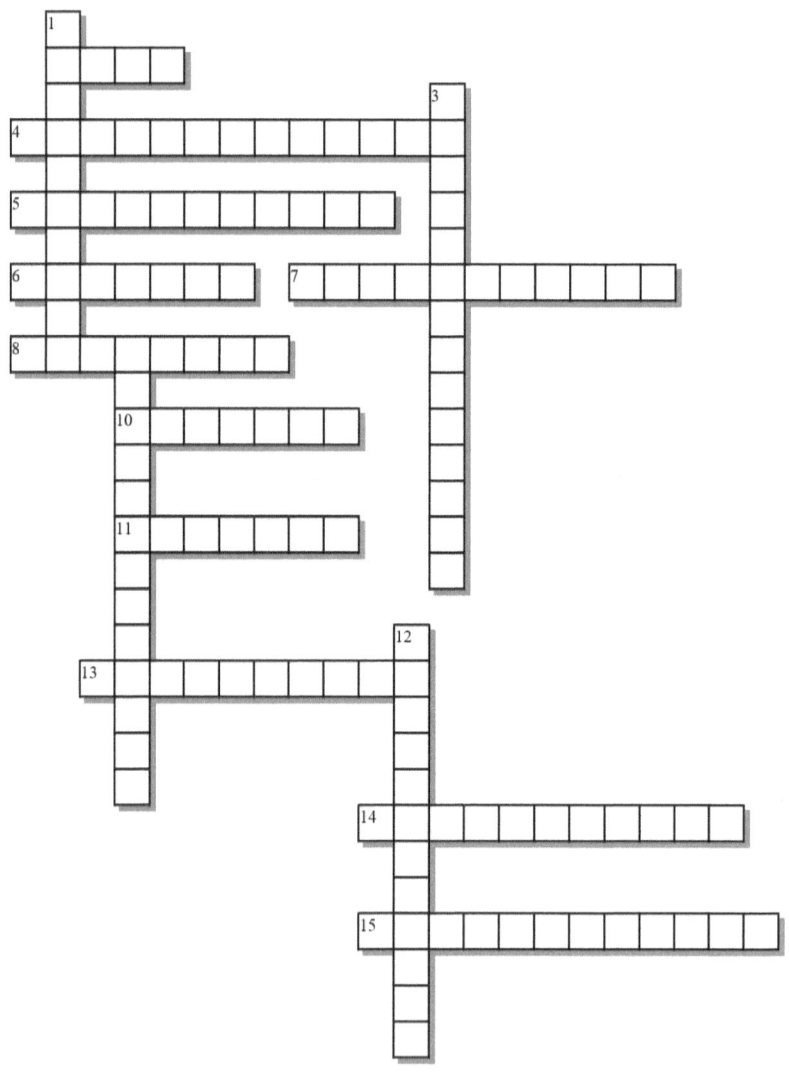

Across:

2 - Brand name for clobetasol foam, used on the scalp

4 - Generic name for Diprosone®

5 - Generic name for Ultravate®

6 - Brand name for OTC hydrocortisone 1% cream, used in itching

7 - Generic name for Cutivate®

8 - Brand name for hydrocortisone valerate

10 - What is the main indication of these topical steroid medications?

11 - Trade name for the tape flurandrenolide

13 - Generic name for Temovate®

14 - Generic name for Florone®

15 - Generic name for Lidex®

Down:

1 - Generic name for Elocon®

3 - Generic name for Topicort®

9 - Generic name for Aristocort® or Kenalog®

12 - Generic name for Derma-Smoothe/FS® oil, used for relief of ear itching

Urinary Incontinence Medications

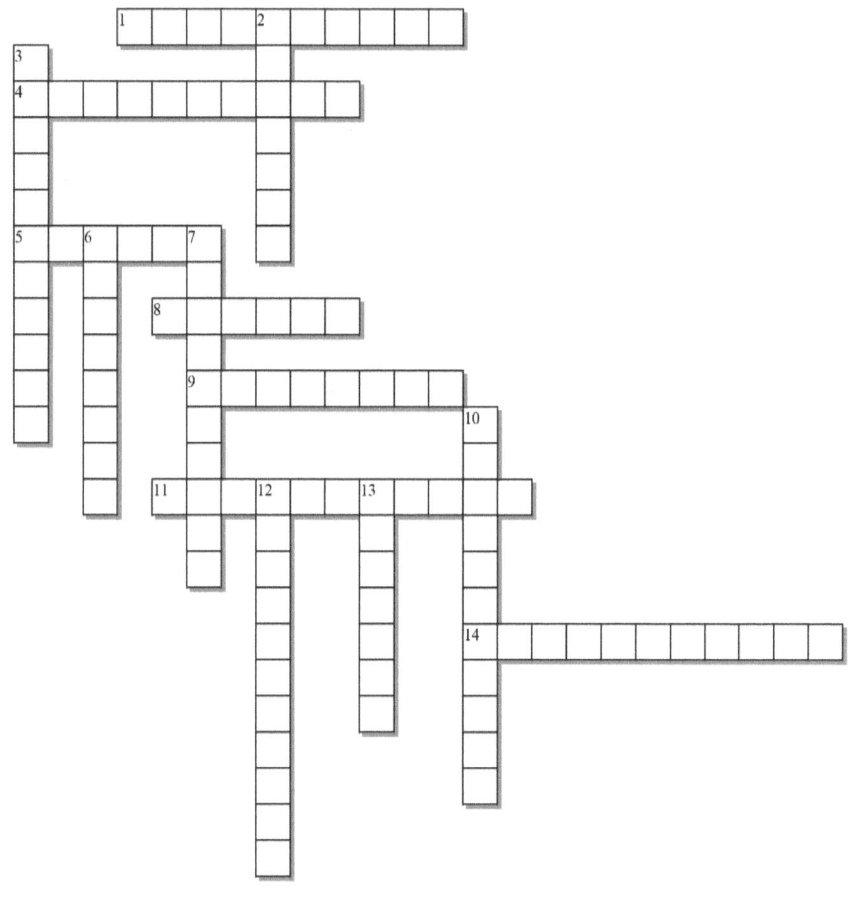

Across:

1 - Generic name for Ditropan®

4 - Generic name for Tofranil®

5 - Trade name for hyoscyamine

8 - Brand name for fesoterodine

9 - Trade name for trospium

11 - Generic name for Urecholine®

14 - Generic name for Detrol®

Down:

2 - Brand name for flavoxate

3 - Generic name for Bentyl®

6 - Trade name for solifenacin

7 - What is the main side effect of these medications used in treating urinary incontinence?

10 - Brand name for propantheline

12 - Generic name for Levsinex®

13 - Brand name for darifenacin

Answers to
Crossword Puzzles
and
Word Search

Angiotensin Converting Enzyme (ACE) Inhibitors

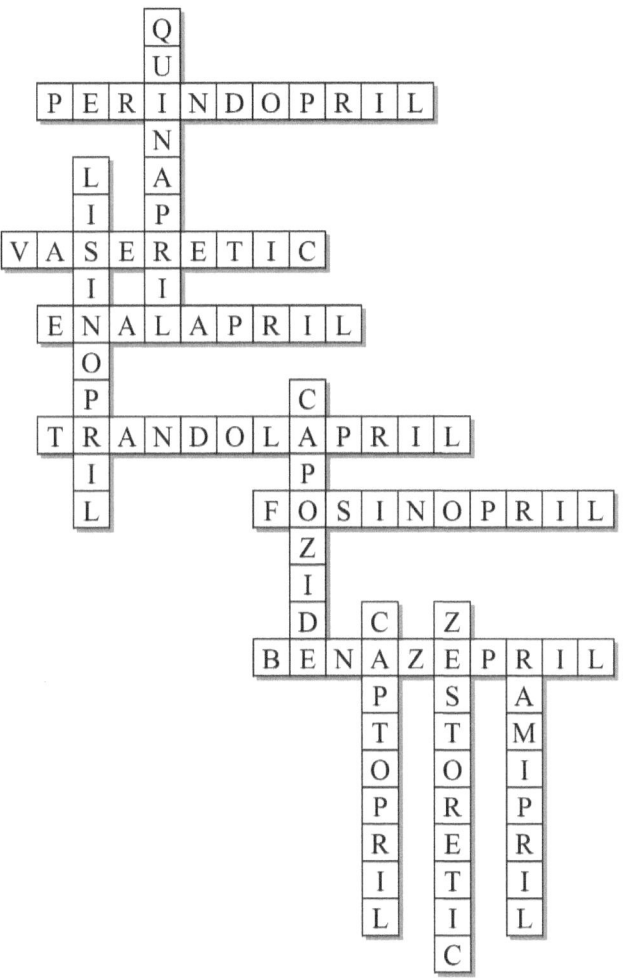

Antiarrhythmic Medications

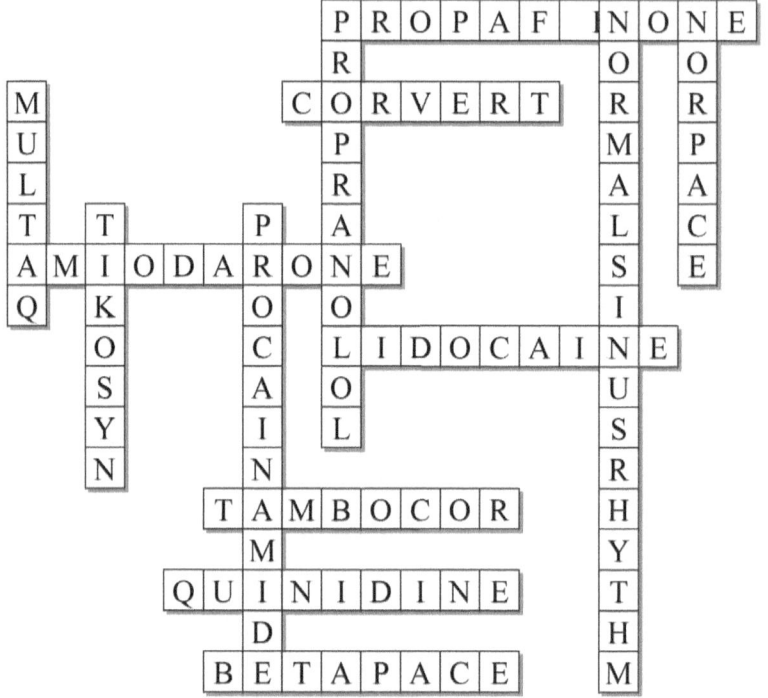

Antibiotics

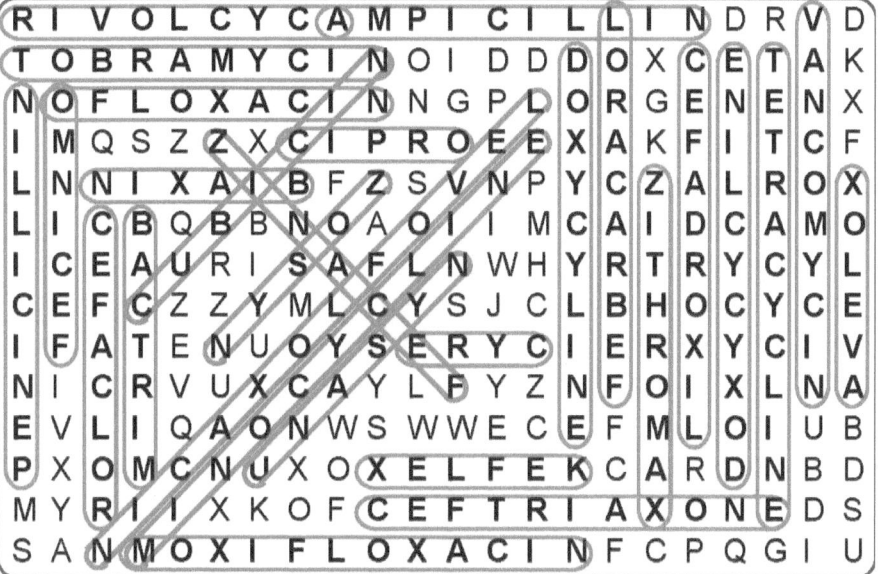

```
R I V O L C Y C A M P I C I L L I N D R V D
T O B R A M Y C I N O I D D D O X C E T A K
N O F L O X A C I N N G P L O R G E N E N X
I M Q S Z Z X C I P R O E E X A K F I T C F
L N N I X A I B F Z S V N P Y C Z A L R O X
L I C B Q B B N O A O I I M C A I D C A M O
I C E A U R I S A F L N W H Y R T R Y C Y L
C E F C Z Z Y M L C Y S J C L B H O C Y C E
I F A T E N U O Y S E R Y C I E R X Y C I V
N I C R V U X C A Y L F Y Z N F O I X L N A
E V L I Q A O N W S W W E C E F M L O I U B
P X O M C N U X O X E L F E K C A R D N B D
M Y R I I X K O F C E F T R I A X O N E D S
S A N M O X I F L O X A C I N F C P Q G I U
```

Anticancer Medications

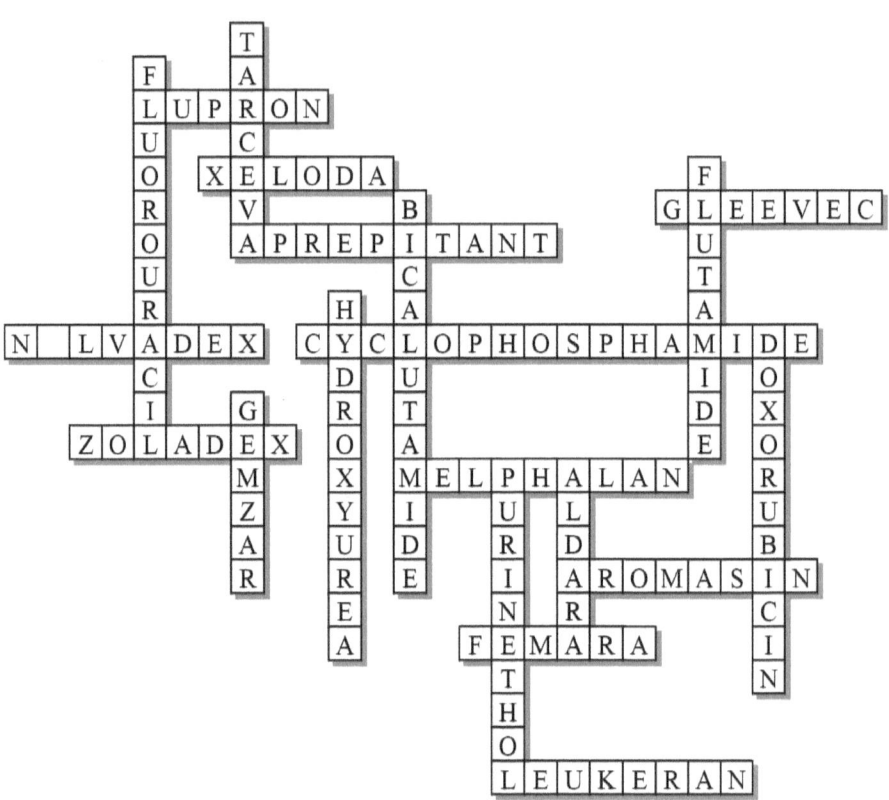

Antidepressant Medications

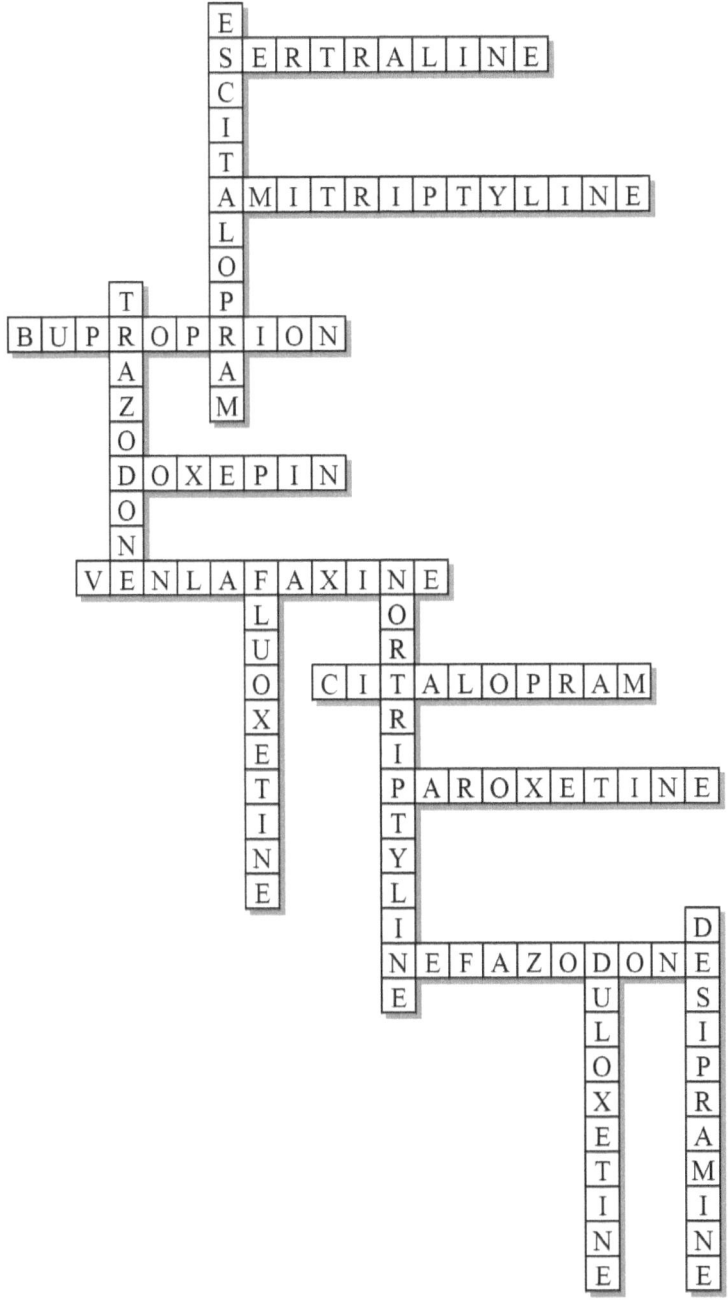

Anti-Drug Category

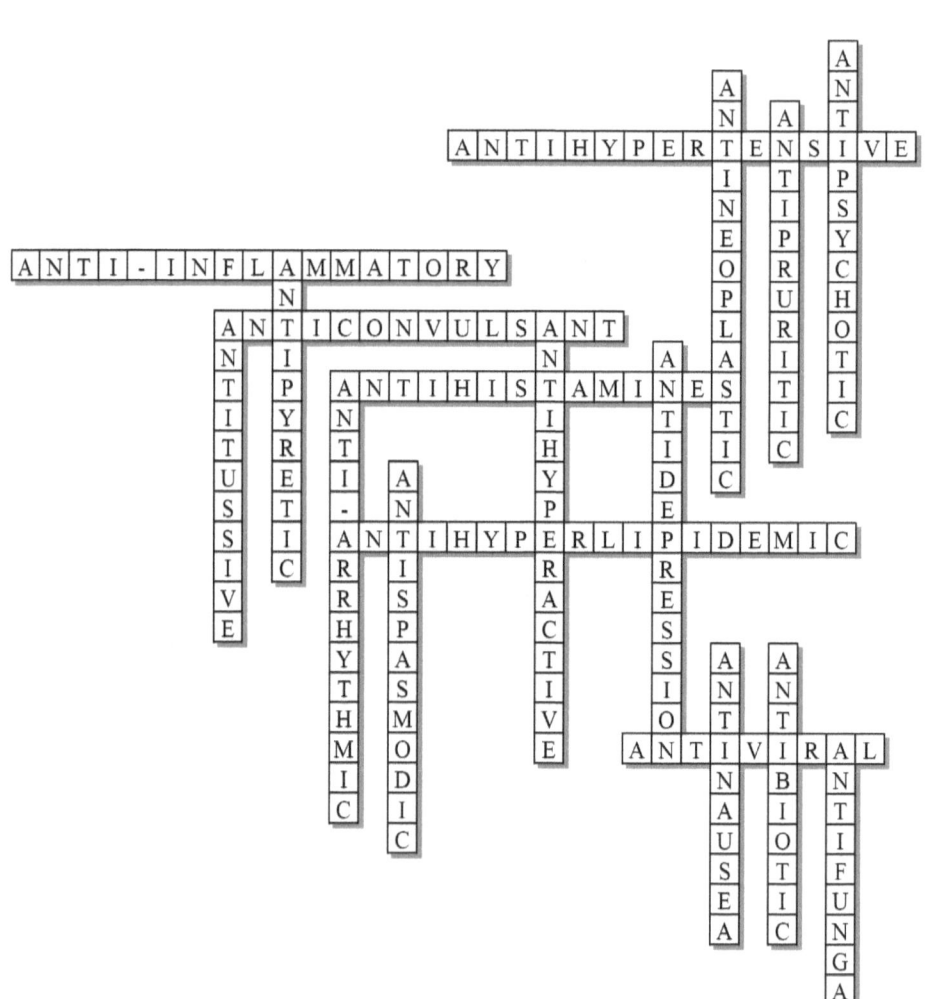

Antifungal Medications

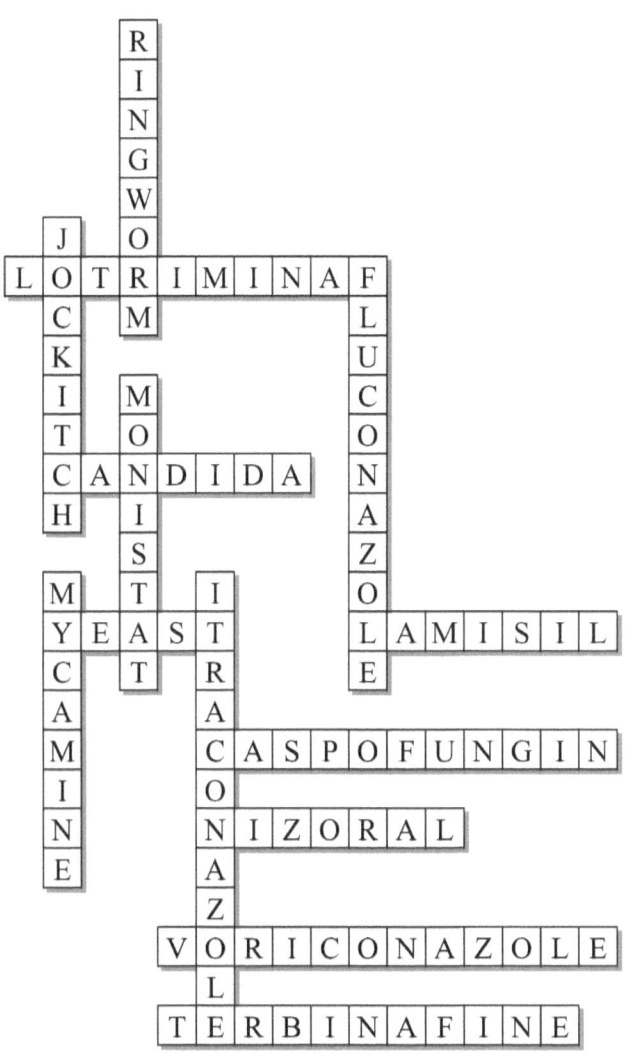

Antihistamines

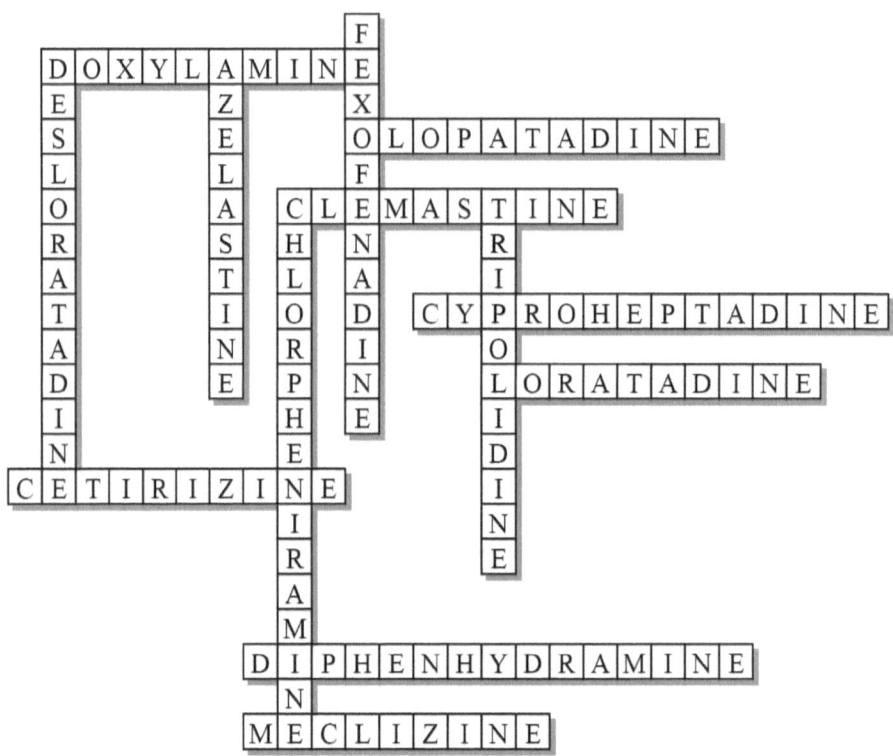

Antihyperlipidemic Medications

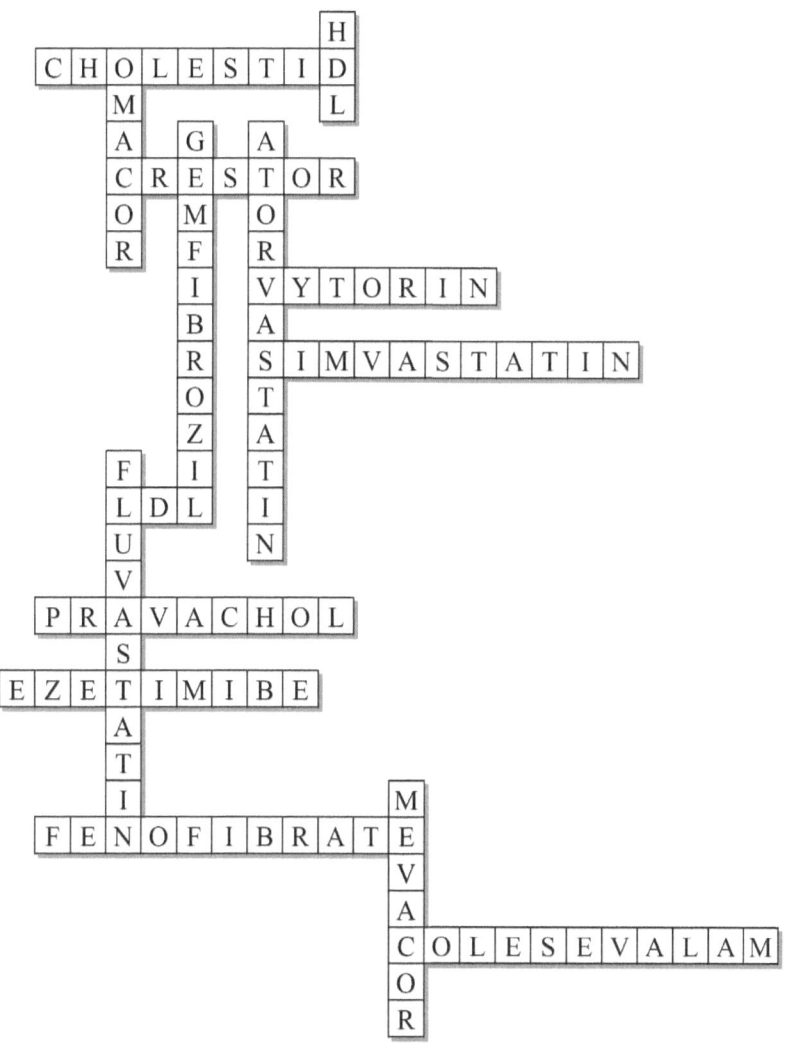

Anti-Parkinson's Medications

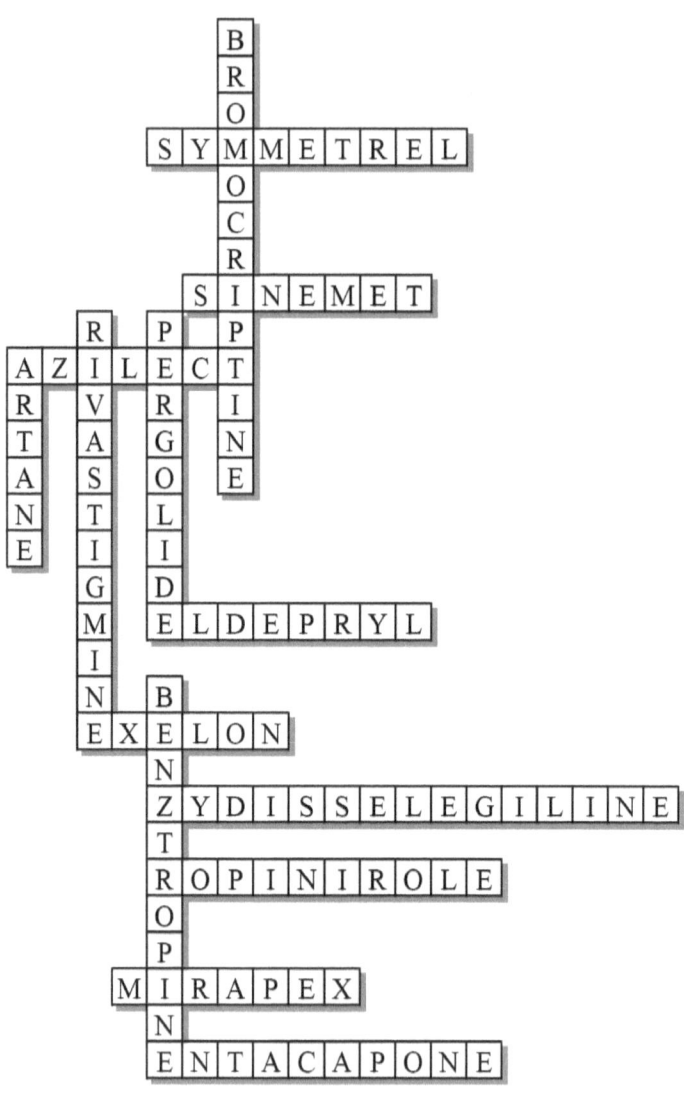

Attention-Deficit/Hyperactivity Disorder Medications

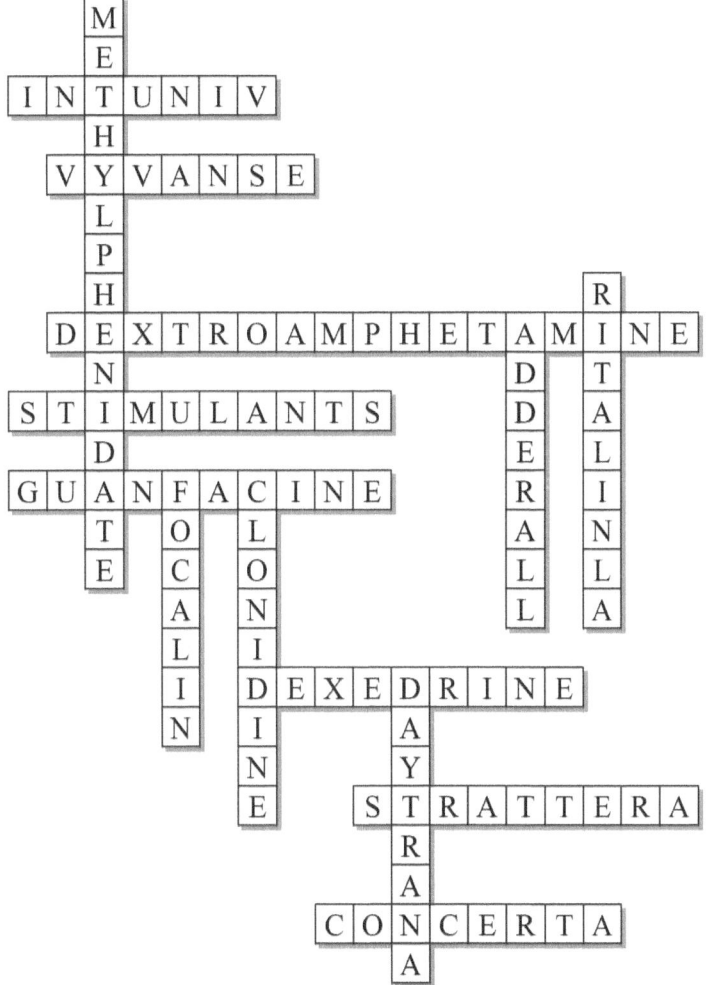

Benzodiazepine Medications

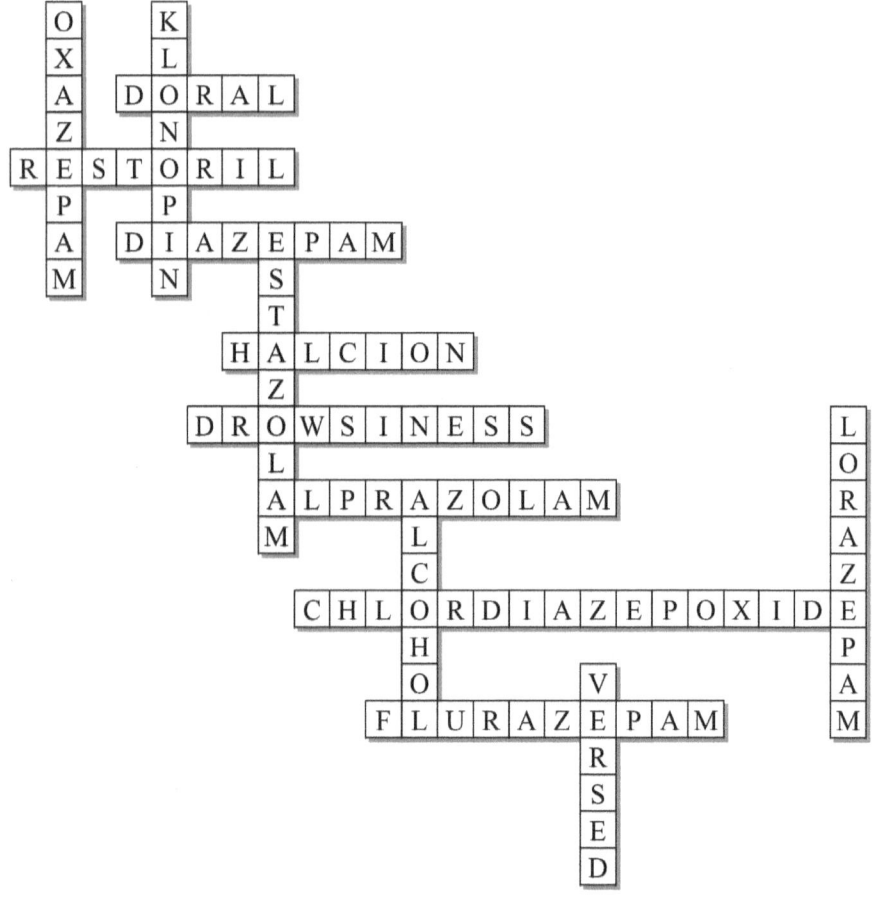

Beta-Blockers Medications

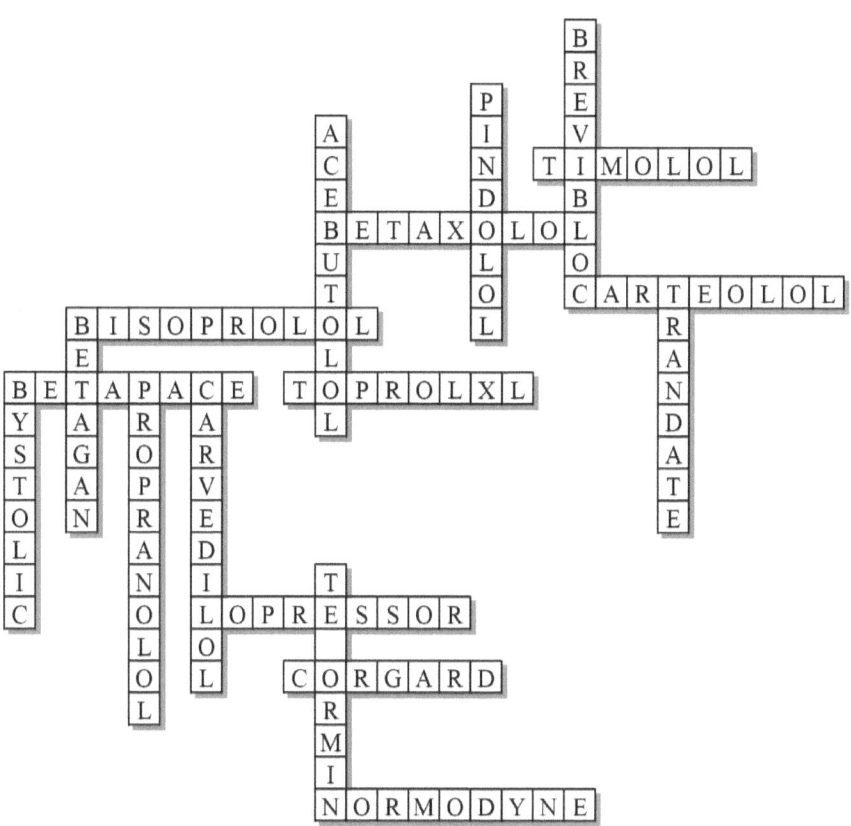

Calcium Channel Blockers

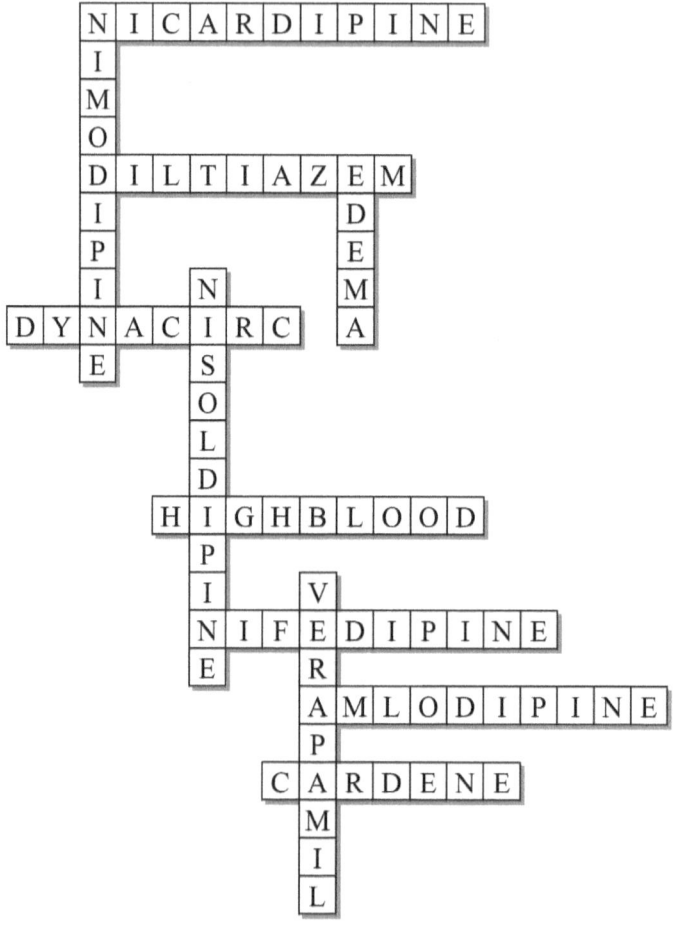

Central Nervous System Medications

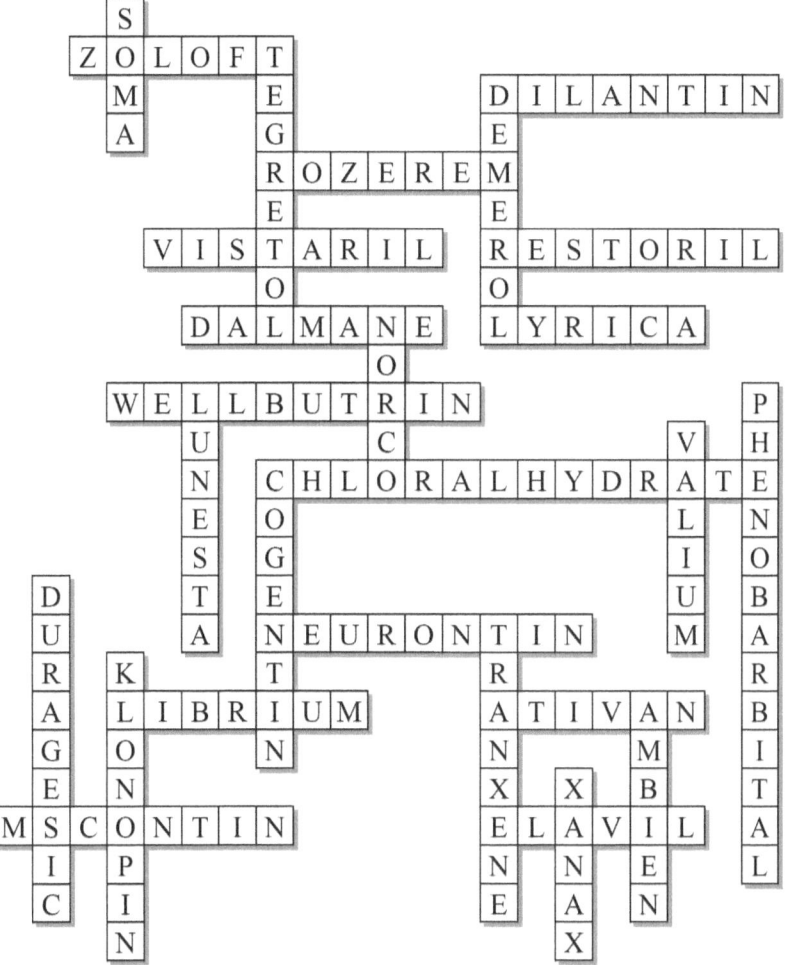

Cephalosporin Antibiotics

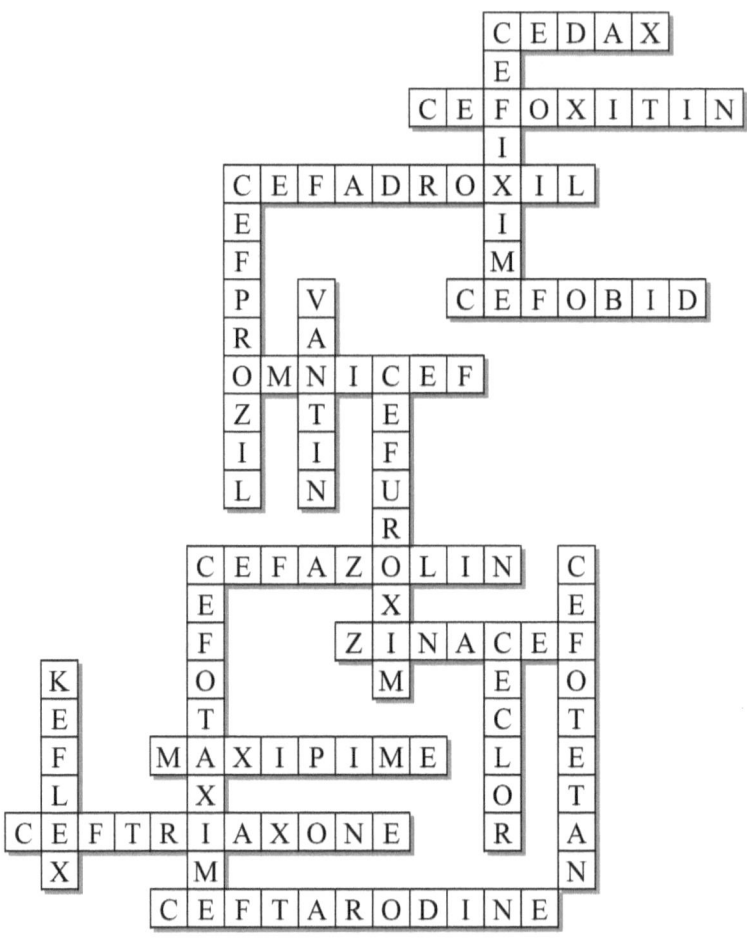

Common Antidotes

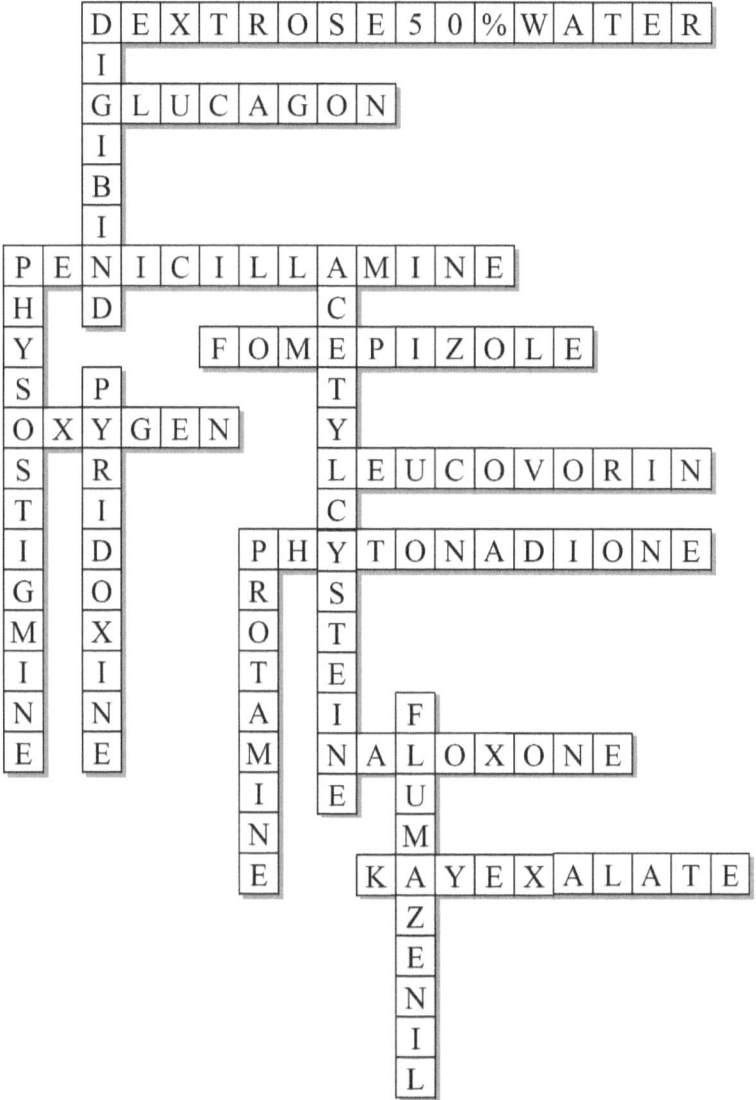

Common Drugs Available in Orally Disintegrating Tablet Forms

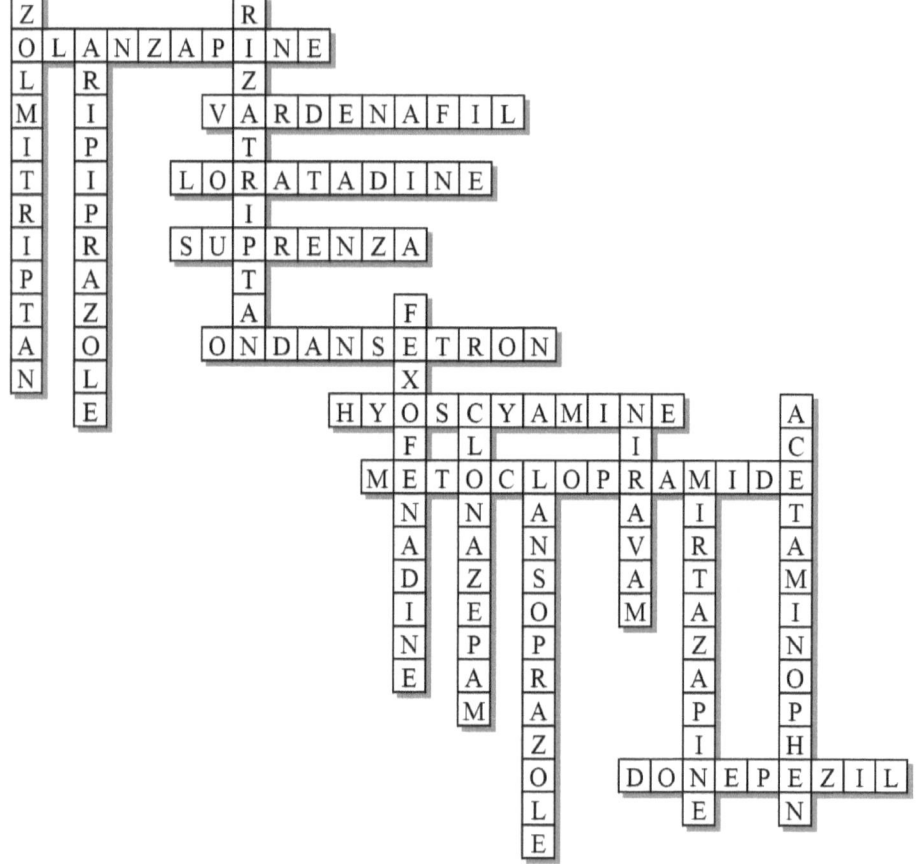

Common Drugs to be Avoided After Gastric Bypass

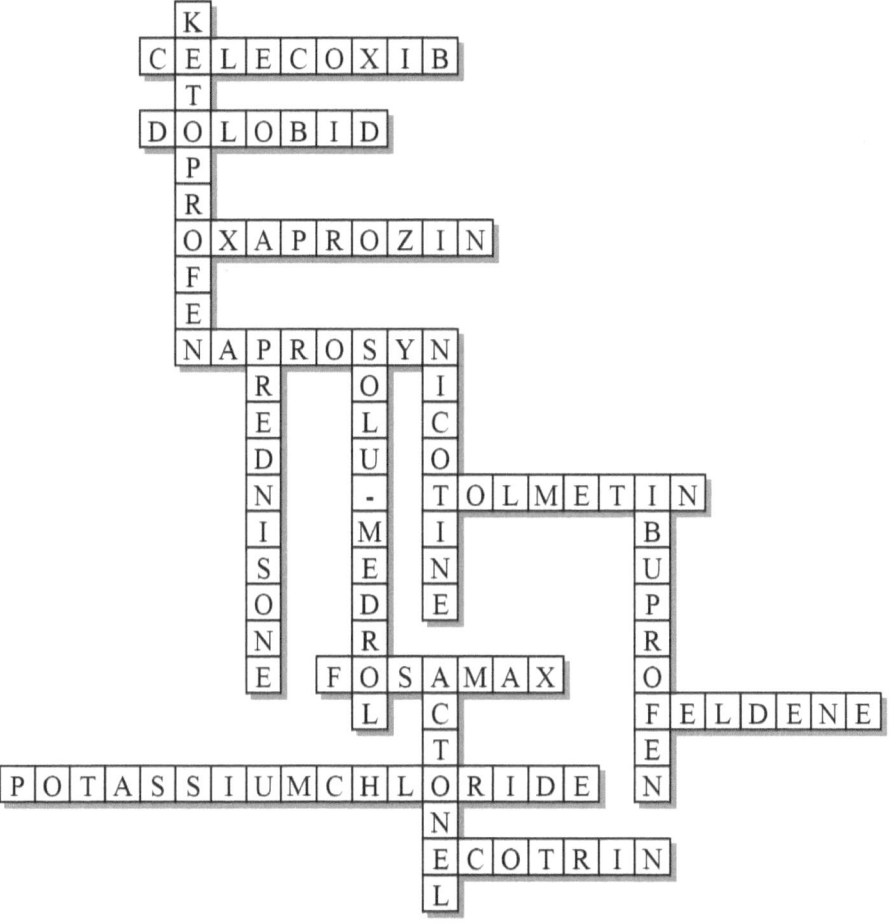

Common Drugs
Used in Blood Transfusion

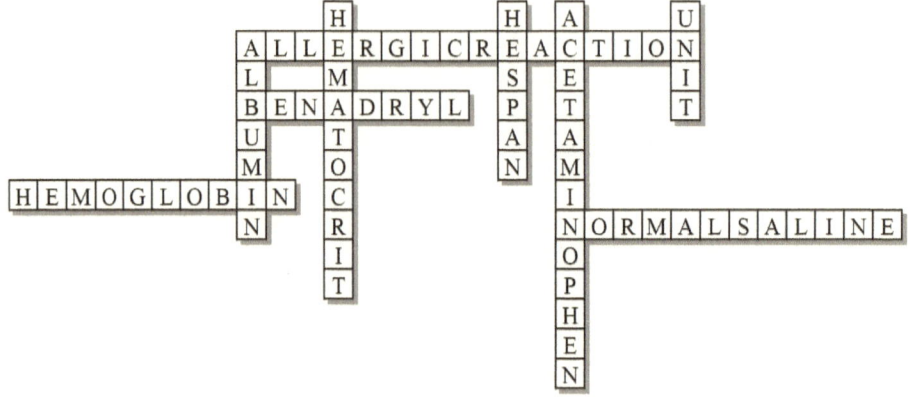

Common Drugs Used in Palliative Care for Comfort Measure

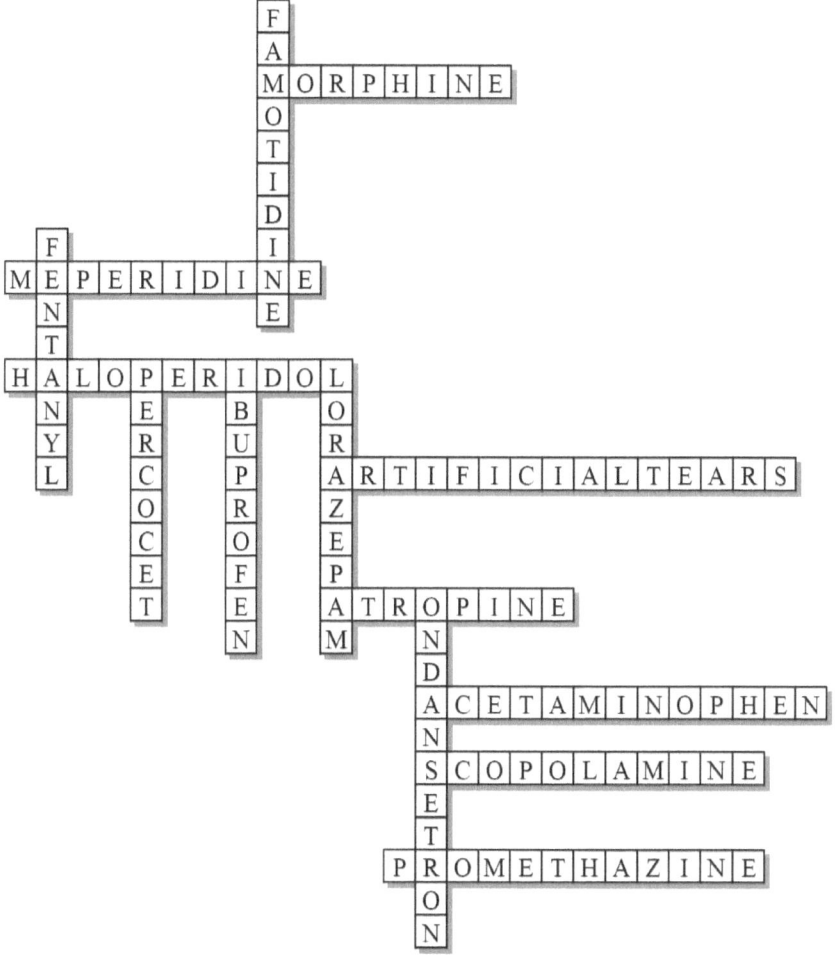

Common Drugs with
Black Box Warnings

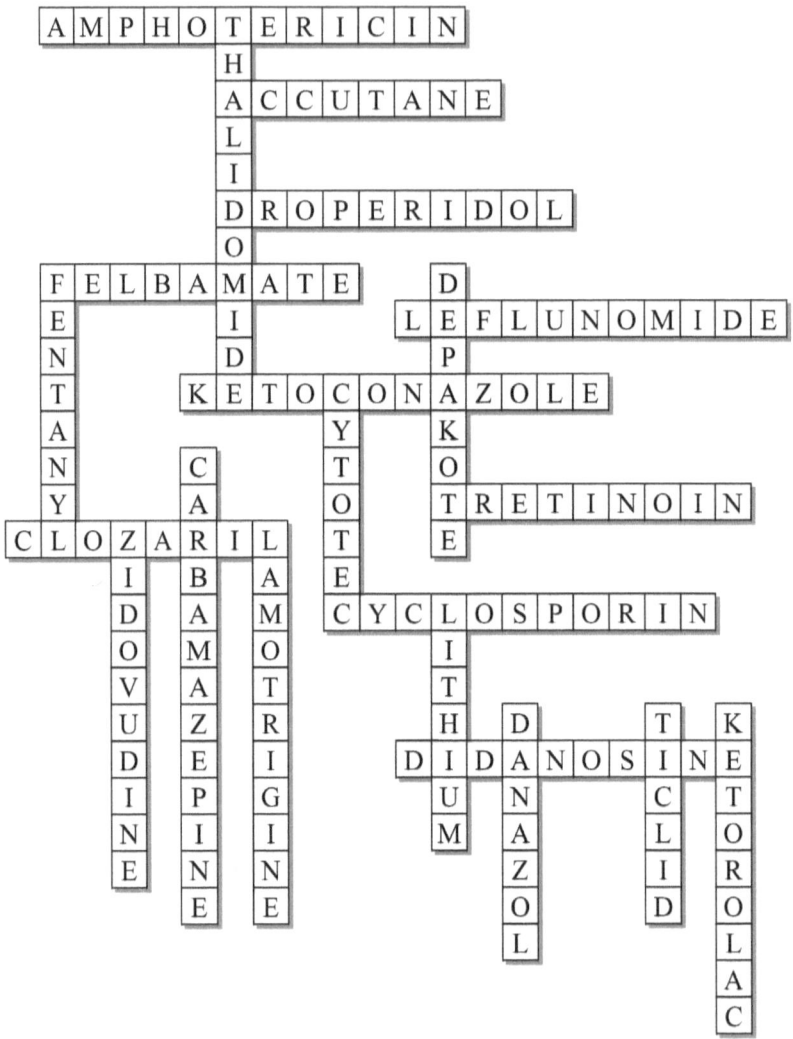

Common Heartburn Medications

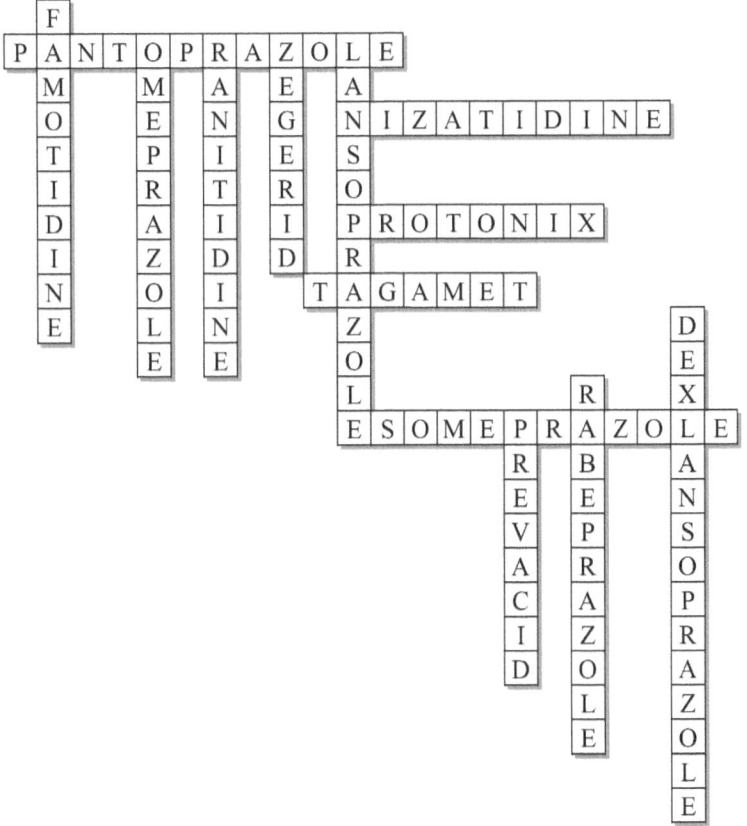

Common Medications
Cannot be Crushed

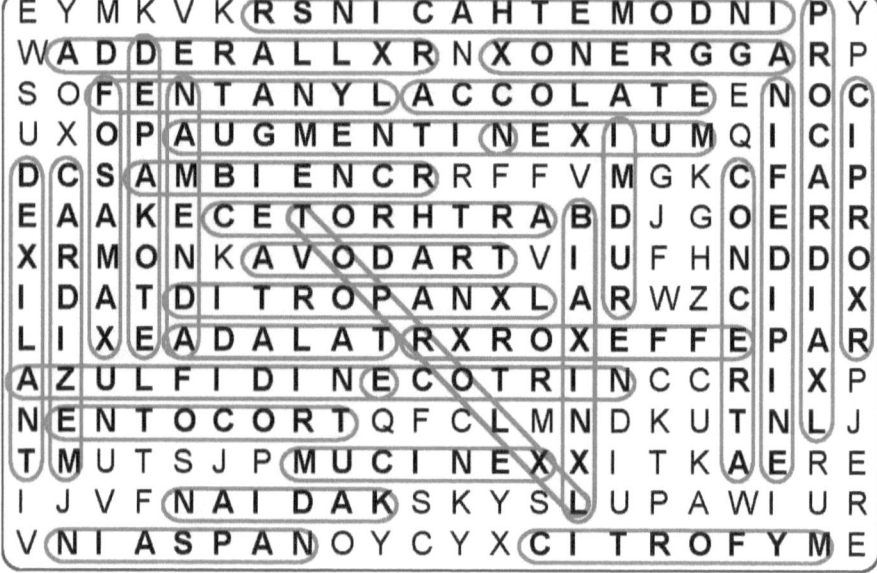

E Y M K V K R S N I C A H T E M O D N I P Y
W A D D E R A L L X R N X O N E R G G A R P
S O F E N T A N Y L A C C O L A T E E N O C
U X O P A U G M E N T I N E X I U M Q I C I
D C S A M B I E N C R R F F V M G K C F A P
E A A K E C E T O R H T R A B D J G O E R R
X R M O N K A V O D A R T V I U F H N D D O
I D A T D I T R O P A N X L A R W Z C I I X
L I X E A D A L A T R X R O X E F F E P A R
A Z U L F I D I N E C O T R I N C C R I X P
N E N T O C O R T Q F C L M N D K U T N L J
T M U T S J P M U C I N E X X I T K A E R E
I J V F N A I D A K S K Y S L U P A W I U R
V N I A S P A N O Y C Y X C I T R O F Y M E

Common Medications
Used in Dialysis

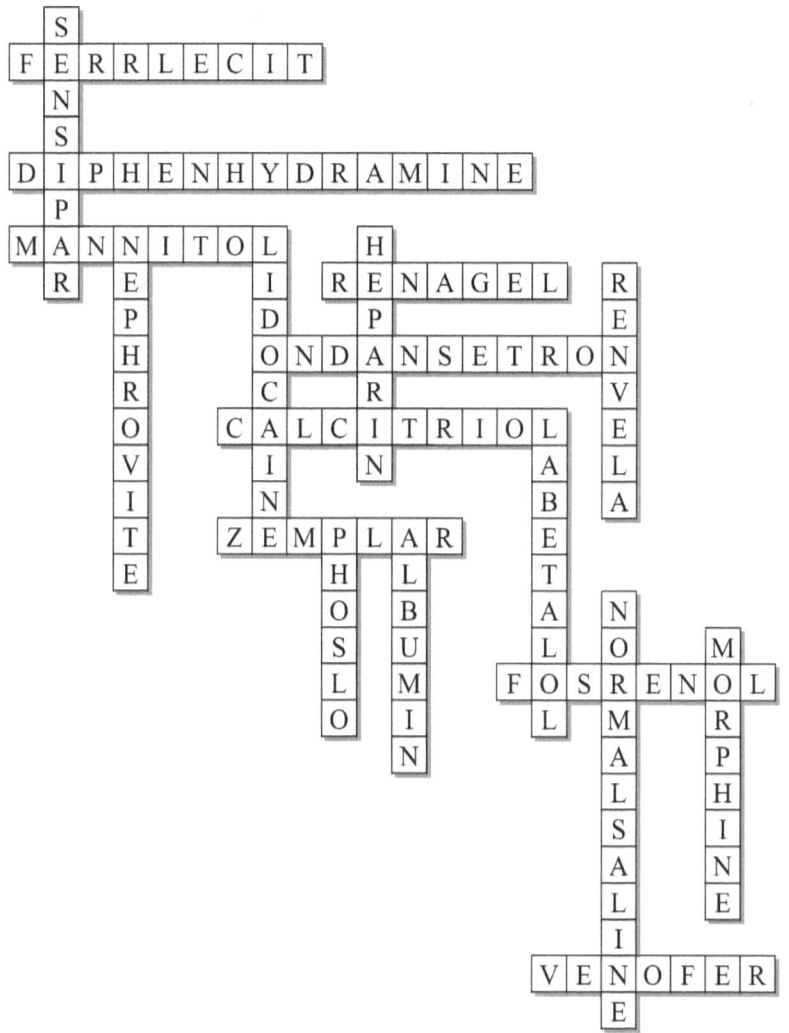

Common Ophthalmic Medications

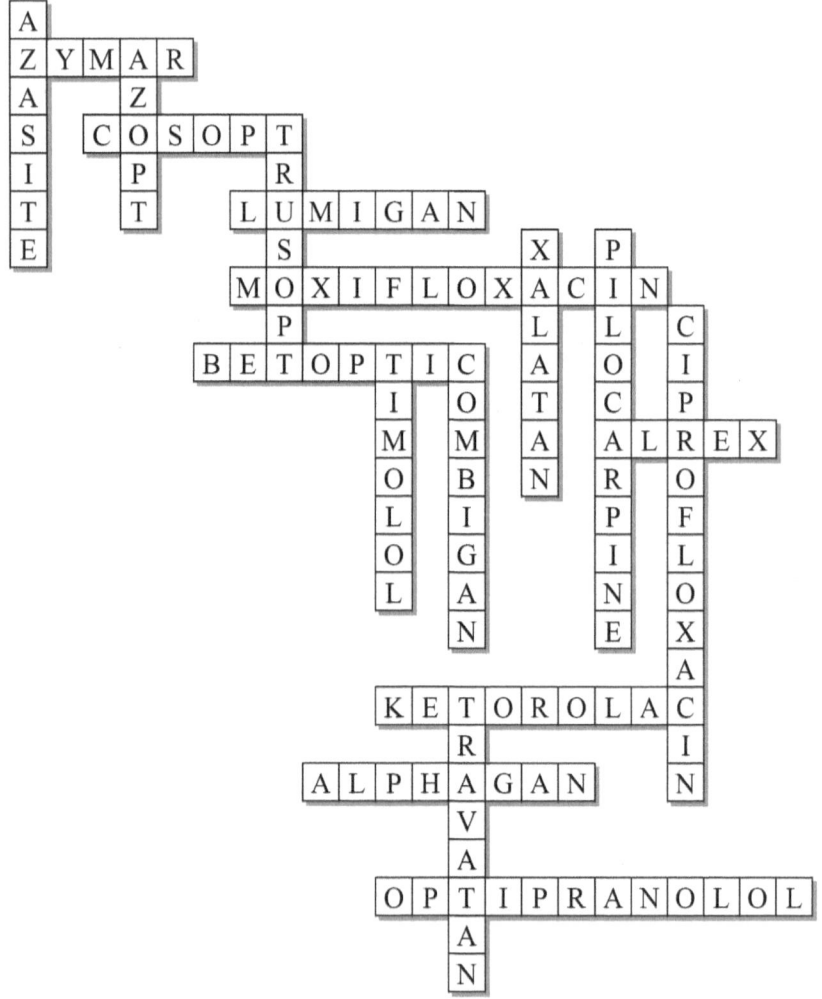

Common Pharmacy References

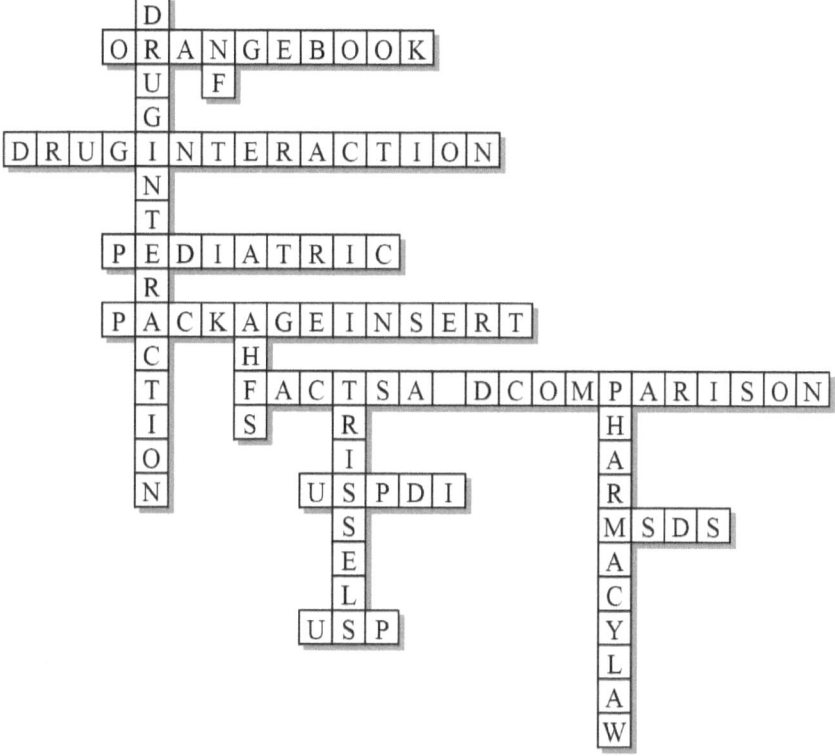

Cytochrome P450 Enzyme Inducers

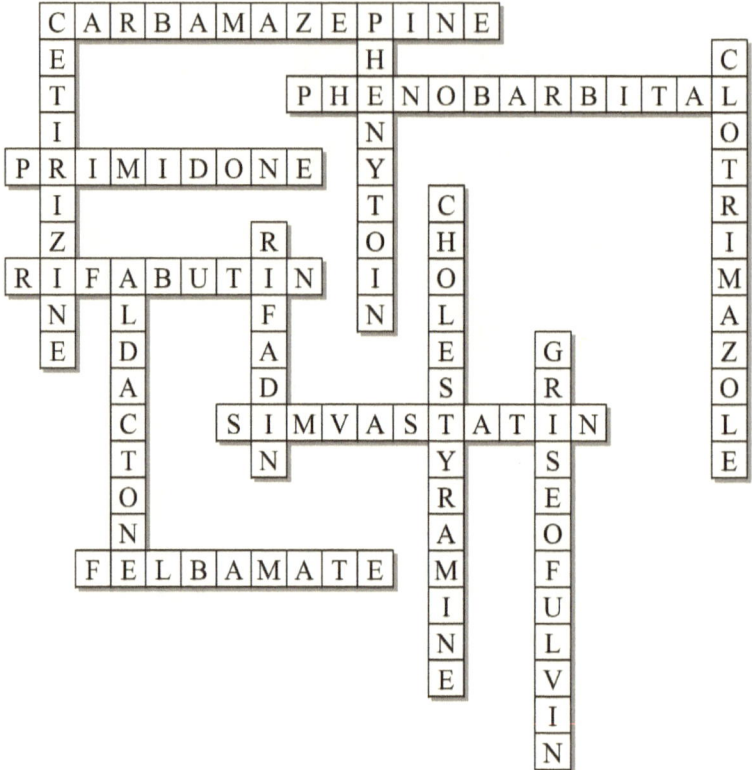

Cytochrome P450
Enzyme Inhibitors

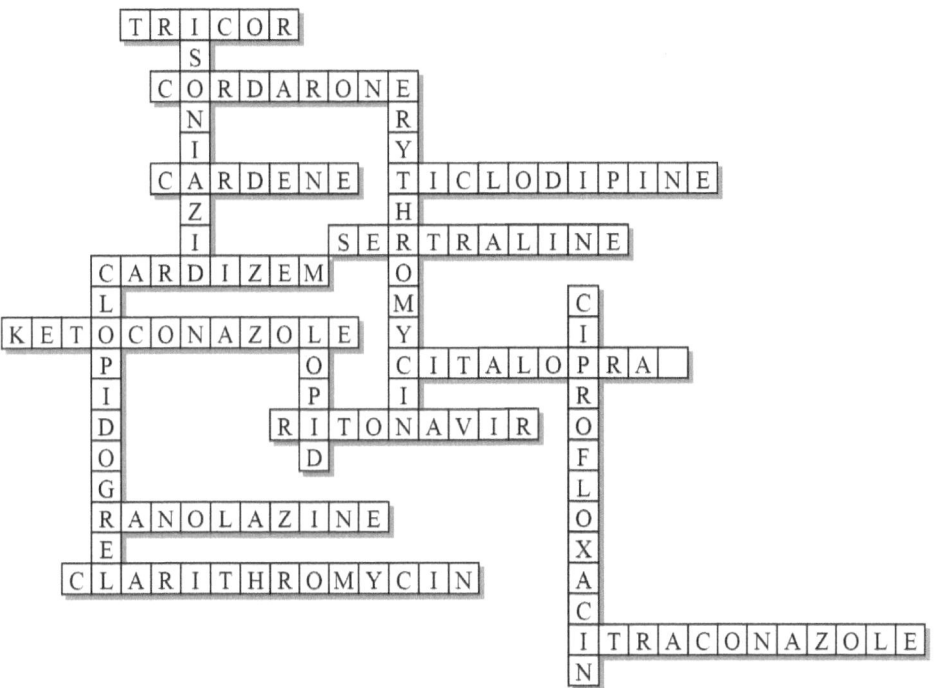

Diabetic Medications
and Supplies

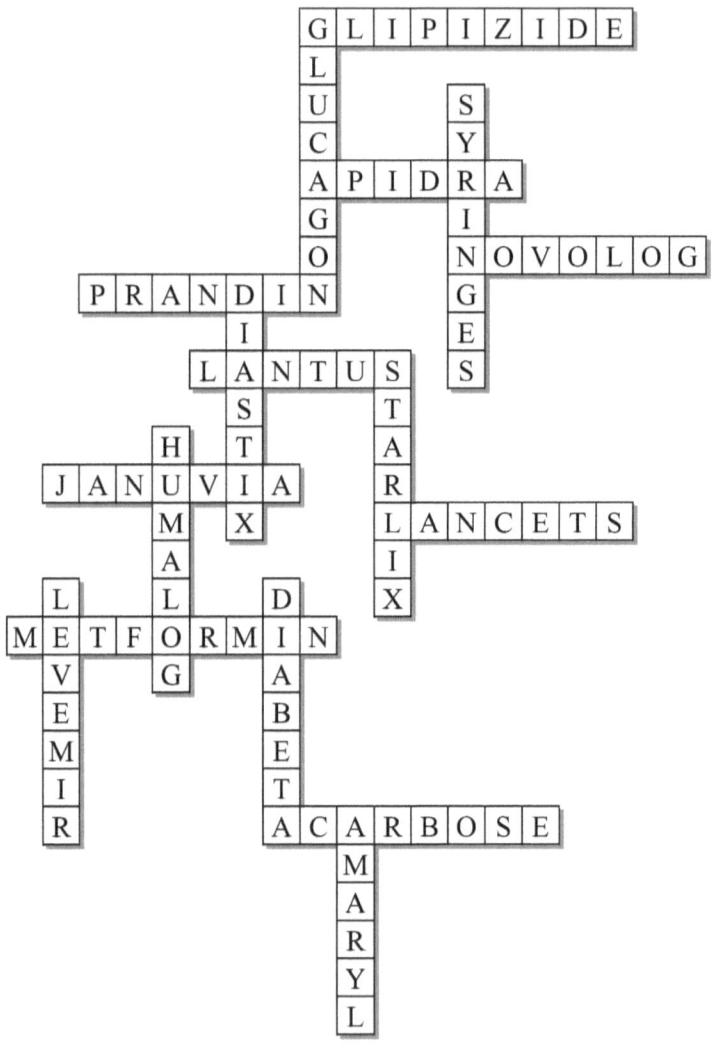

Different Practice Sites

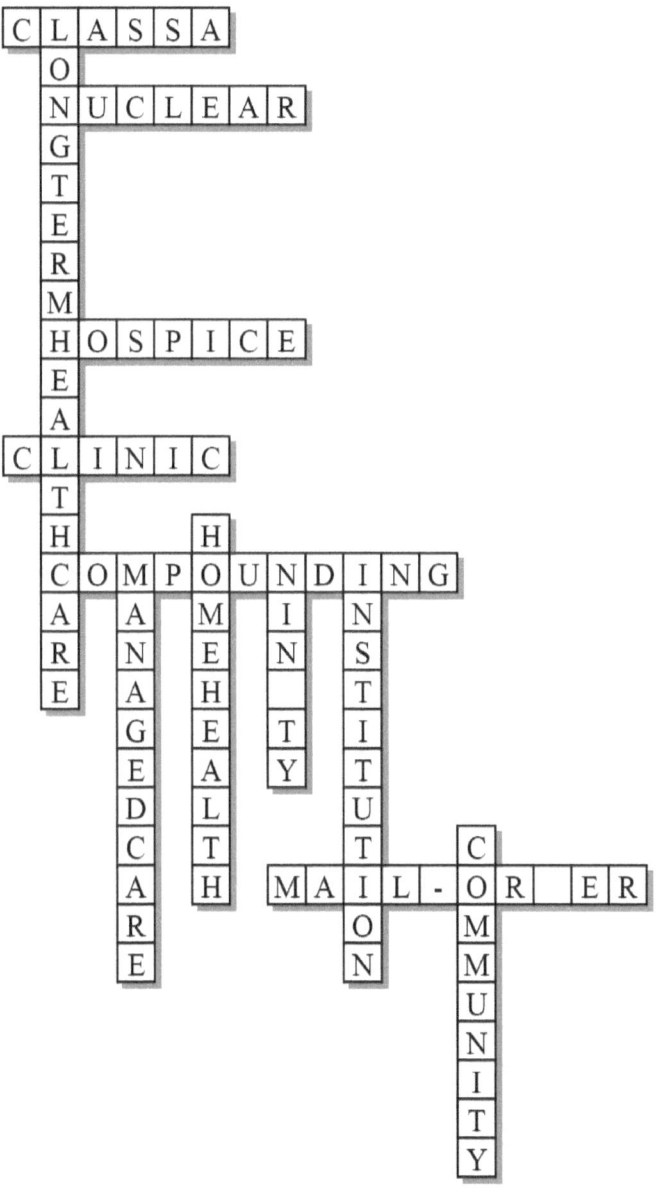

Different Routes of
Administration

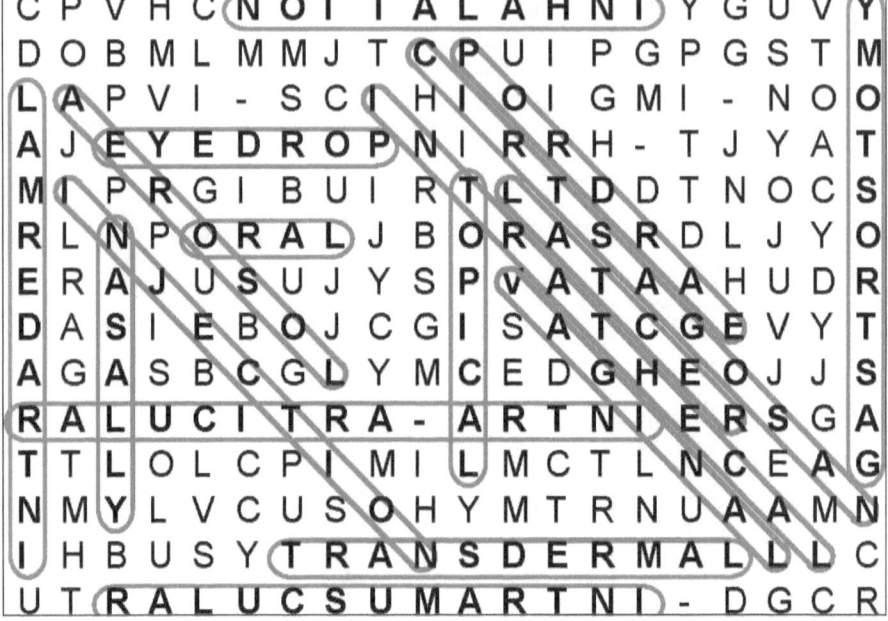

Different Types of
Dosage Form

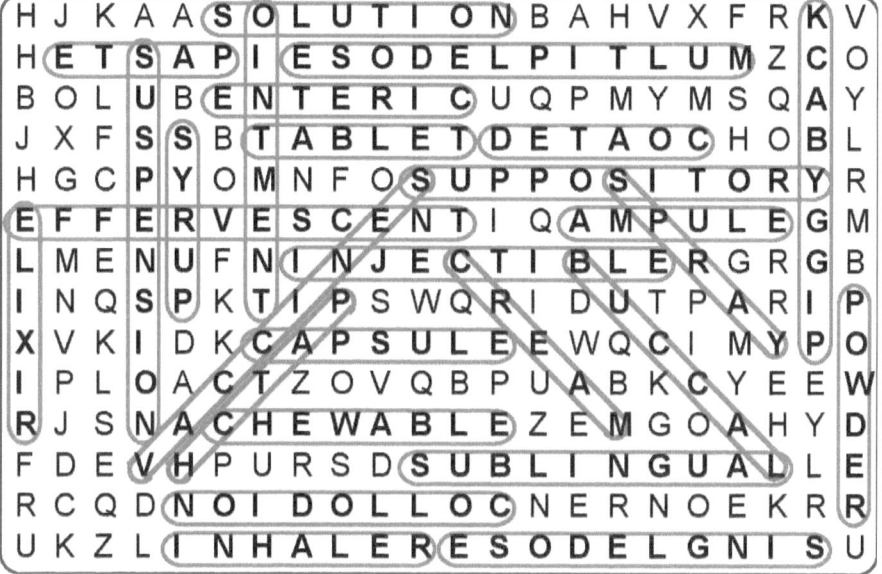

Different Types of Vaccines

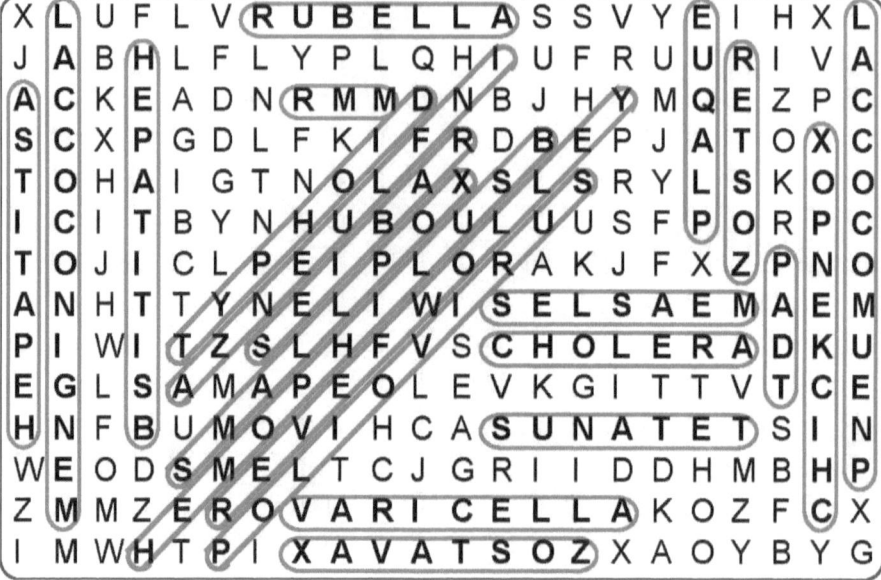

Drugs that Commonly Interact with Grapefruit Juice

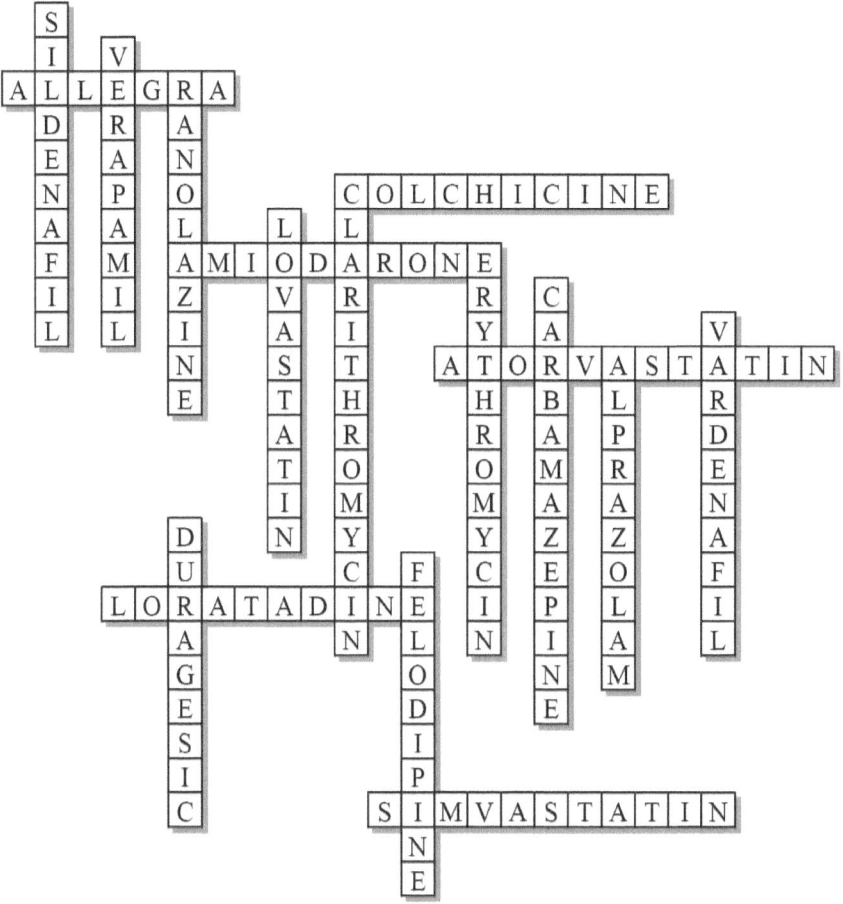

Ear Drops Medications

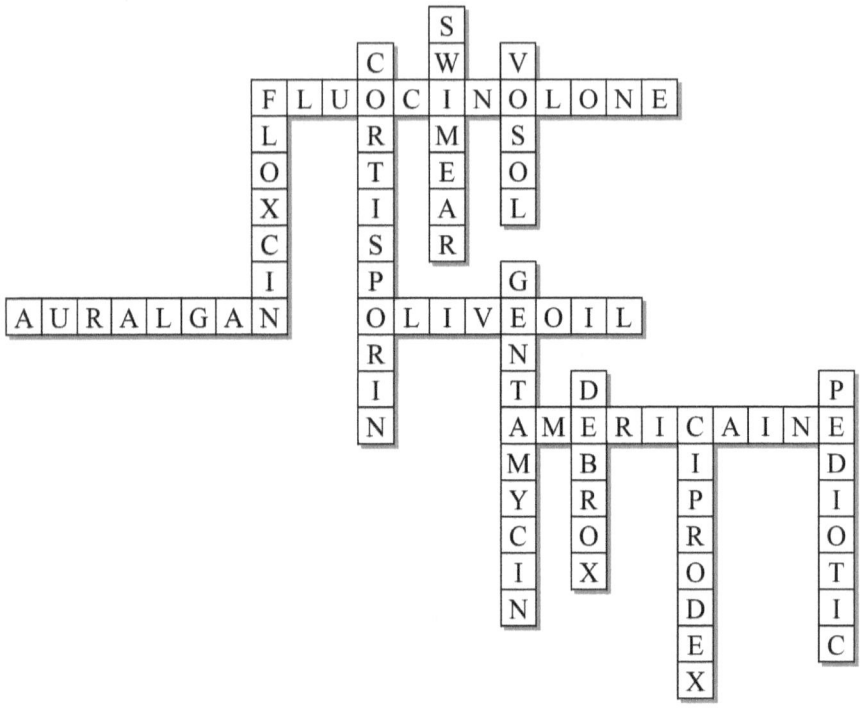

Hormone Medications

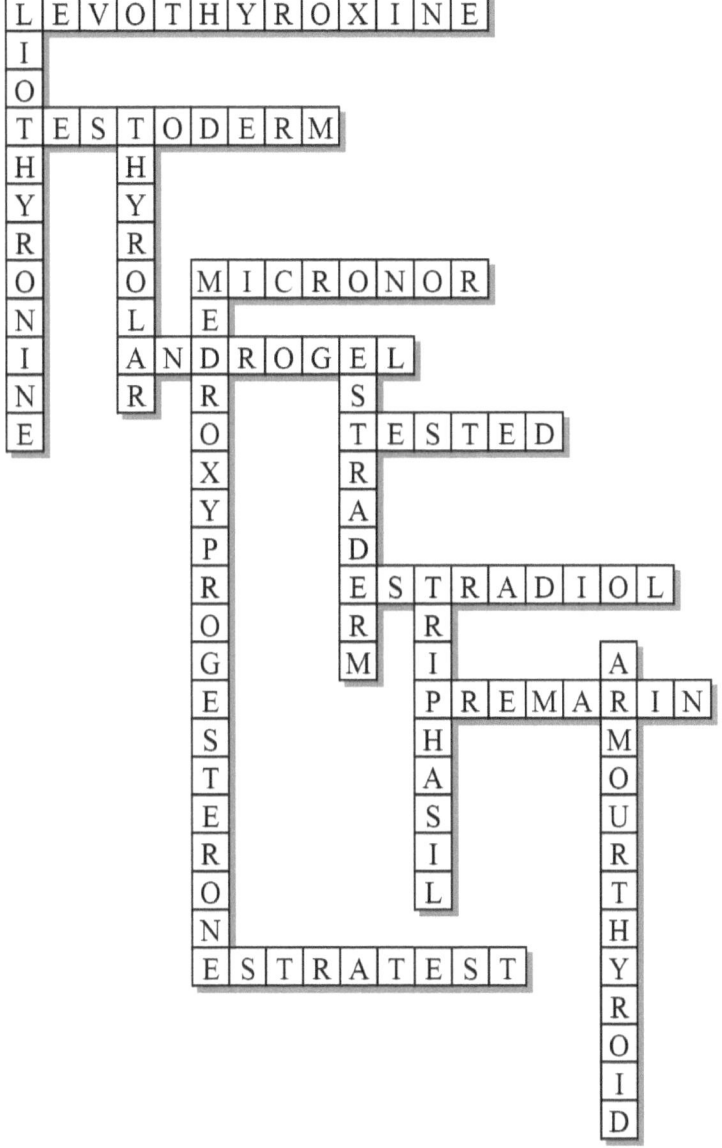

Human Immunodeficiency Virus (HIV) Medications

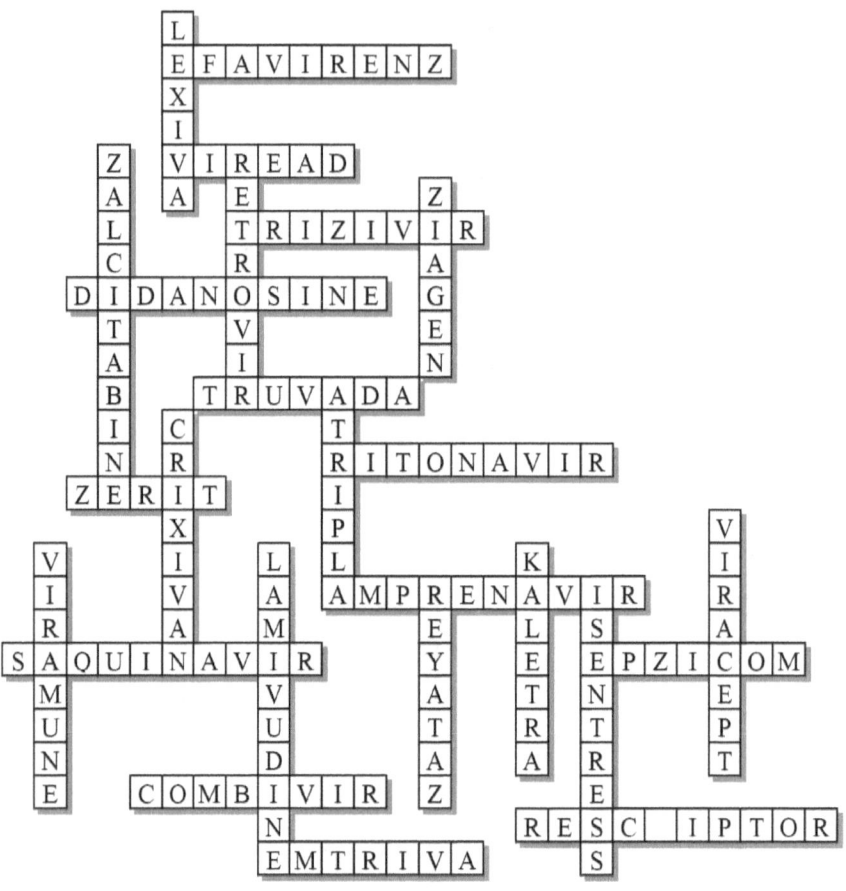

Intravenous Medications
that Require In-line Filters

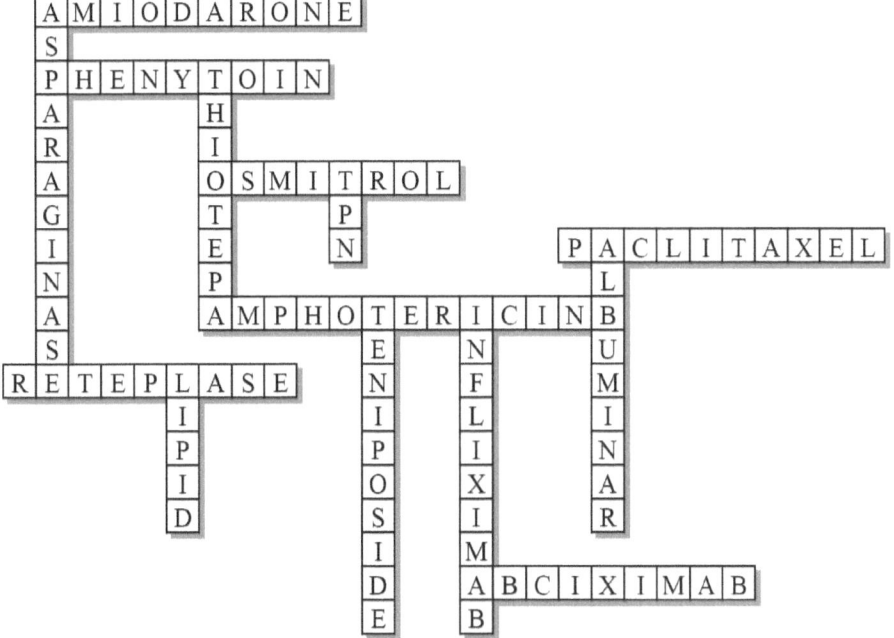

Nonsteroidal Anti-inflammatory Drugs

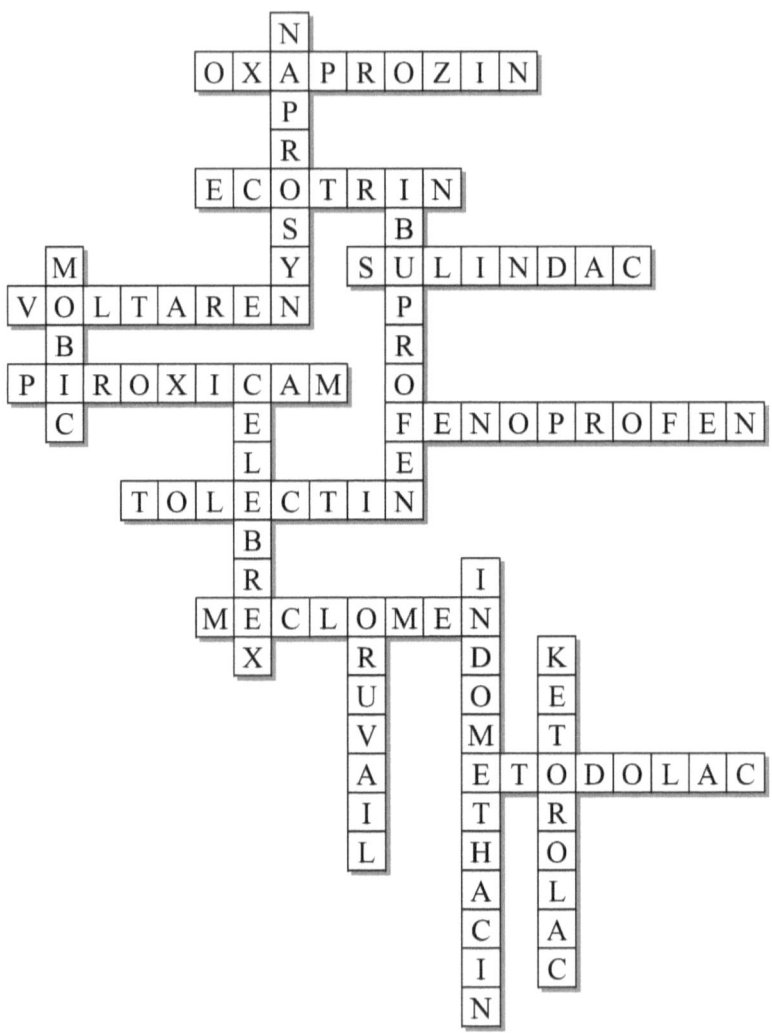

Osteoporosis Medications

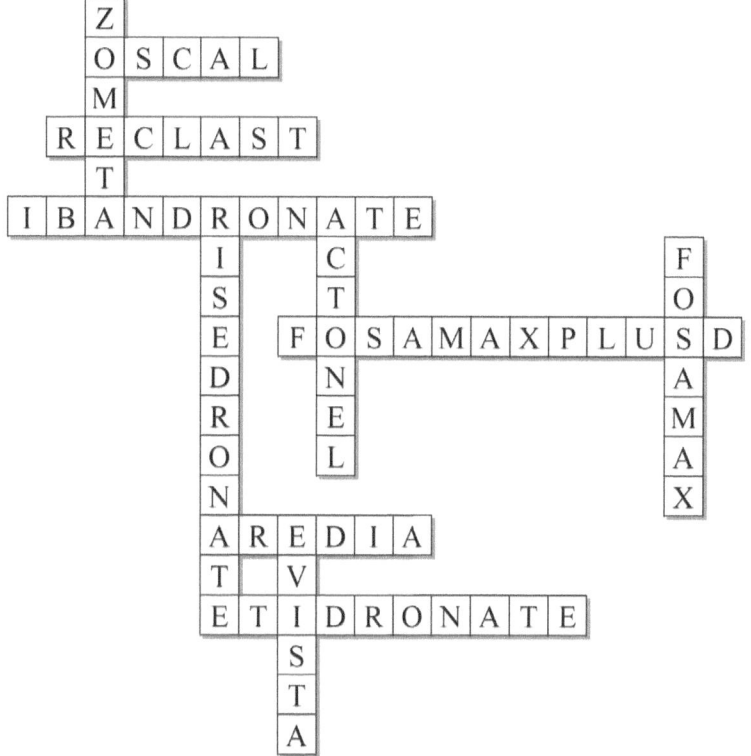

Over-the-Counter
Medications

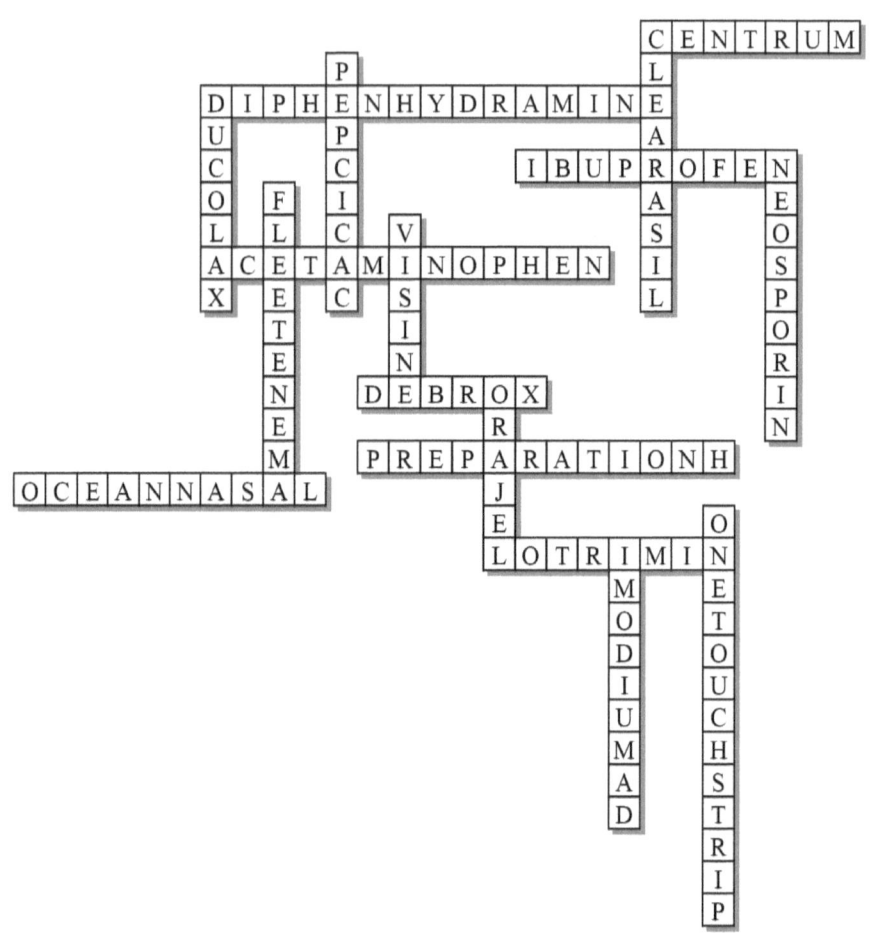

Pain Medications
(Narcotic)

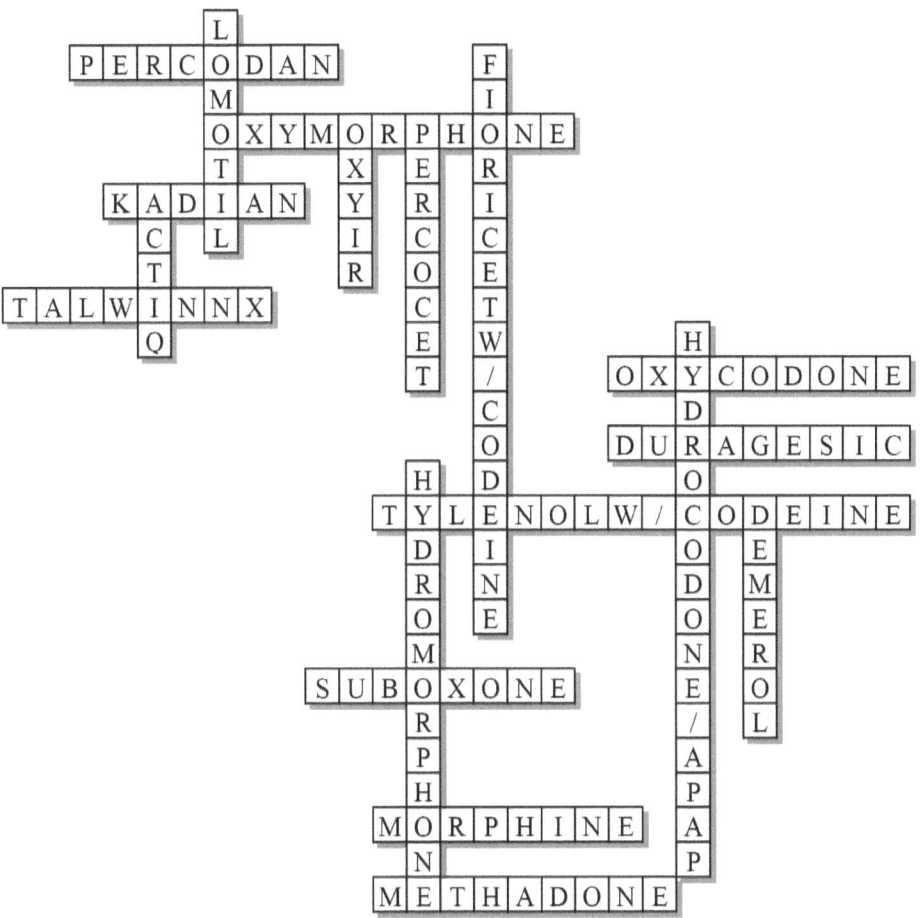

Pain Medications
(Non-narcotic)

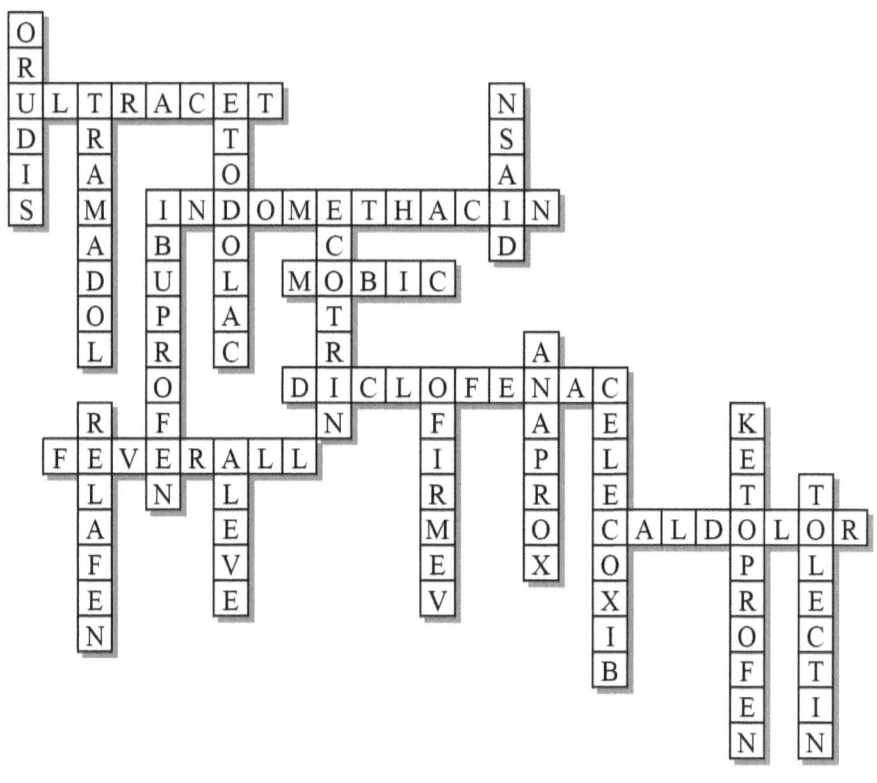

Penicillin and Cephalosporin Antibiotics

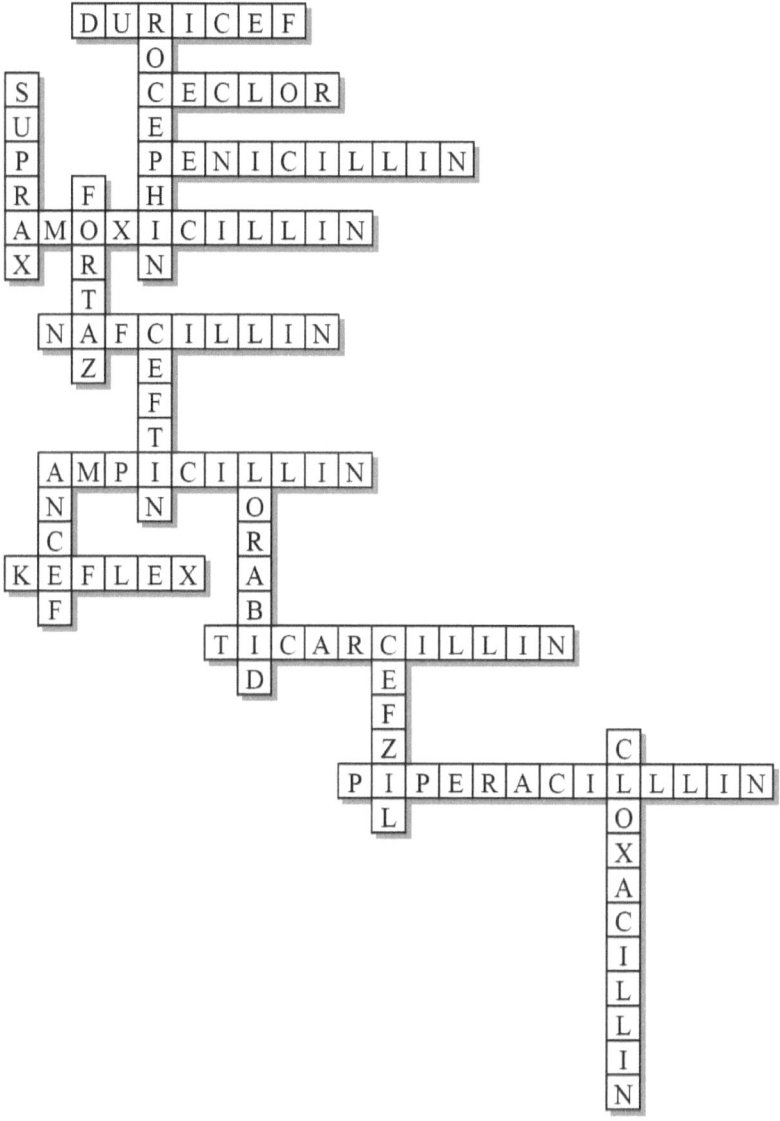

Pharmacy
Health Insurance Review

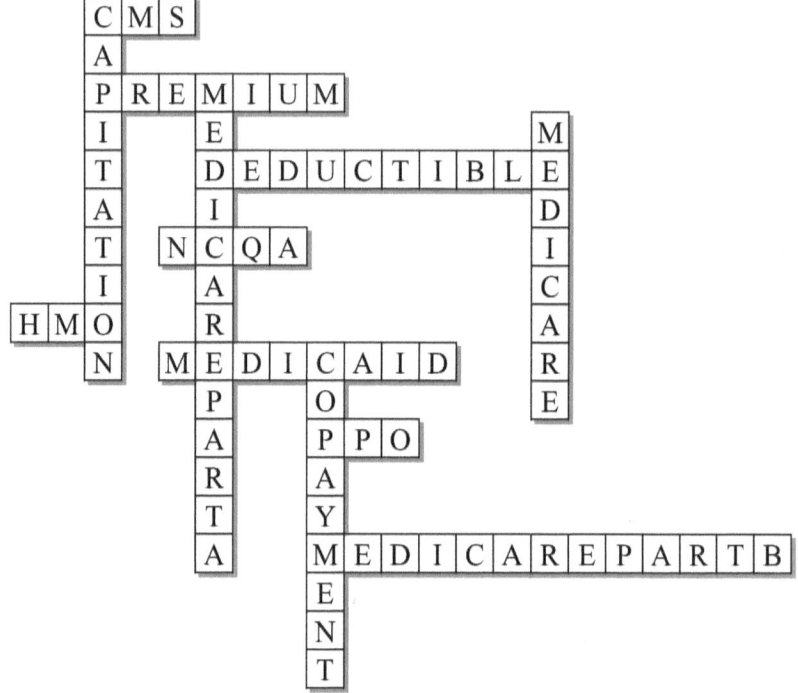

Pharmacy Technician Duties

A S E P T I C T E C H N I Q U E

P R E S C R I P T I O N

B R A N D N A M E   P A T I E N T I N F O R M A T I O N

G E N E R I C

I N V E N T O R Y

N A R C O T I C   C O N S U L T A T I O N

C E R T I F I E D T E C H N I C I A N

R E F I L L

Down words:
- EXPIRATIONDATA
- THIRDPARTY
- COMPUTER
- COPAY
- PRINGENEBOOK
- BRA
- THERAPEUTICSUBSTITUTION
- OVER-THE-COUNTER

Respiratory Medications

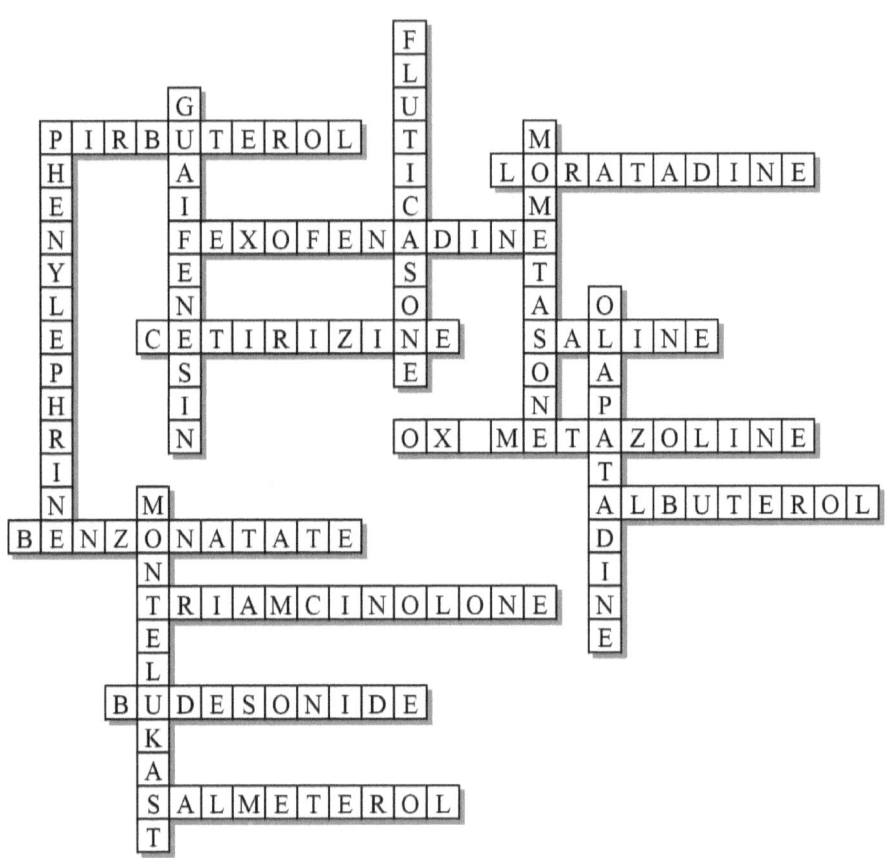

Topical Acne Medications

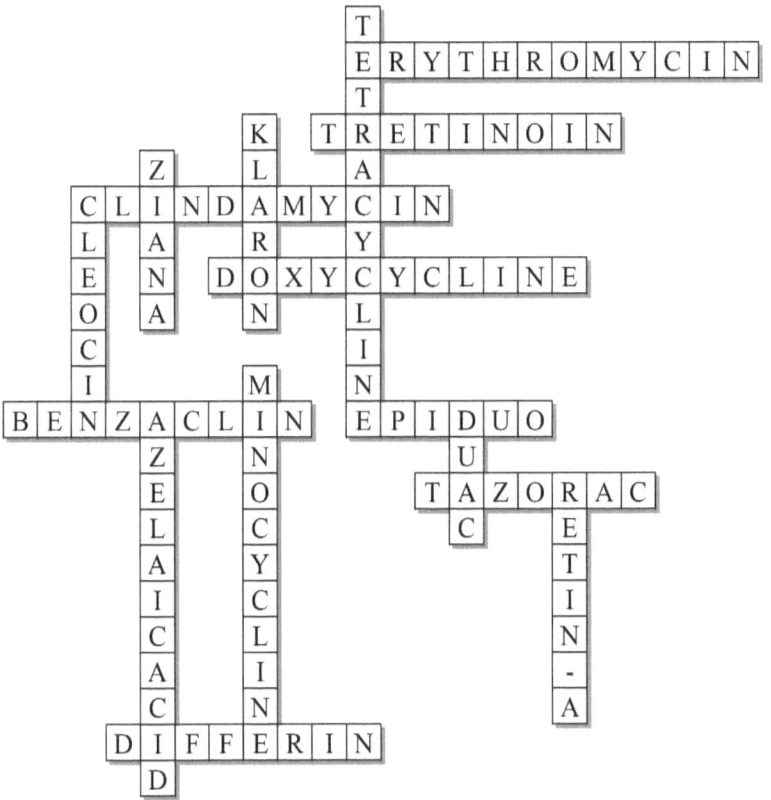

Topical Steroids

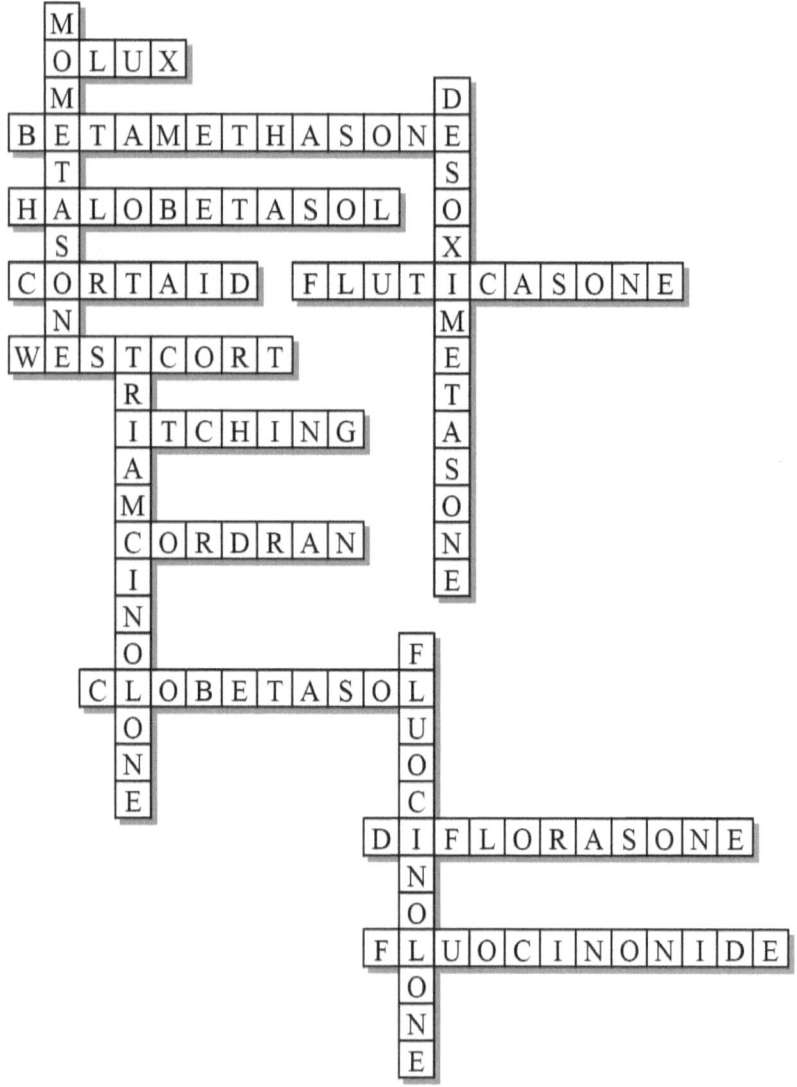

Urinary Incontinence Medications

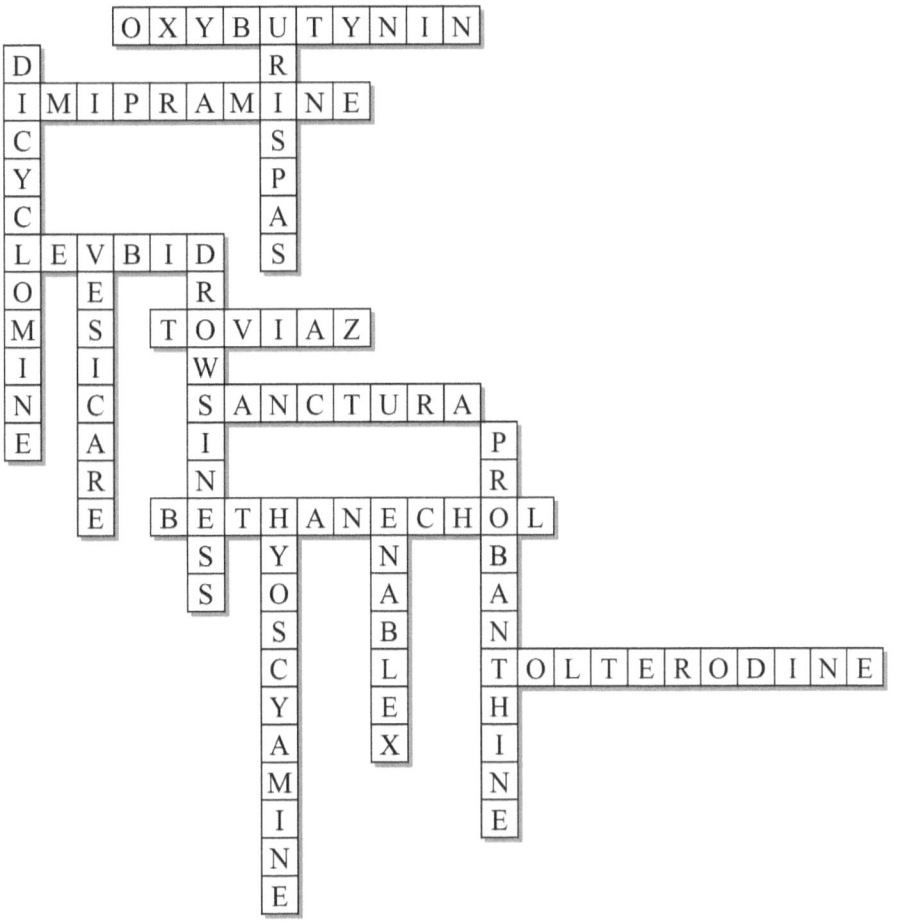

References

Bauer, L. 2008. *Applied Clinical Pharmacokinetics*. 599-619.

DiPiro, J. and B. Wells. 2006. "Dermatologic Disorders." Pharmacotherapy Handbook. 6th Ed. 159-164.

http://www.bariatriceating.com/2011/09/18/list-of-medications-to-avoid-after-gastric-bypass-surgery/ (accessed February 6, 2013).

http://www.emedicinehealth.com/drug-mannitol/article_em.htm (accessed March 1, 2013).

http://www.med.umkc.edu/em/resources/IV_Med_Reference.pdf (accessed February 8, 2013).

http://www.medicinenet.com/thiotepa-injection/article.htm (accessed March 2, 2013).

http://www.pharmacistnewsletter.com (accessed February 15, 2013).

http://www.pharmacologyweekly.com/content/pages/medications-herbs-cytochrome-p450-cyp-enzyme-inhibitors (accessed February 8, 2013).

http://www.pharmacologyweekly.com/content/pages/medications-herbs-cytochrome-p450-cyp-inducers (accessed February 6, 2013).

http://www.pharmacypracticenews.com (accessed February 14, 2013).

http://www.pharmacypracticenews.com/download/BB1044_nexterone_WM.pdf (accessed February 10, 2013).

http://pharmacy.uams.edu/PNP/policy%20507.htm (accessed February 9, 2013).

http://www.pppmag.com/article/353/February_2008/Premixed_IV_ Products/ (accessed February 12, 2013).

http://www.reopro.com/Pages/index.aspx (accessed February 6, 2013).

http://www.healthcare.gov/using-insurance/medicare-long-term-care/ long-term-care/ (accessed February 8th, 2013)

http://www.rxlist.com/cardene-iv-drug.htm (accessed February 14, 2013).

http://www.rxlist.com/elspar-drug.htm (accessed February 15, 2013).

http://www.rxlist.com/fungizone-drug/patient-images-side-effects.htm (accessed March 2, 2013).

http://www.rxlist.com/remicade-drug.htm (accessed March 1, 2013).

http://www.rxlist.com/taxol-drug.htm (accessed February 19, 2013).

http://www.rxlist.com/vumon-drug.htm (accessed February 19, 2013).

http://www.utmb.edu/rxhome/Operations/Filtrations.htm (accessed February 8, 2013).

Kasper, D. and A. Fauci. 2010. *Harrison's Infectious Diseases*. 275-282.

Lacy, C., Armstrong, L., Goldman, M. and L. Leonard, eds. 2011-2012. *Lexi-Comp's Drug Information Handbook: A Comprehensive Resource for All Clinicians and Healthcare Professionals*. 20th Ed. 102-113, 580-585, 987, 1187, 1247, and 1683.

McElroy, G. et al. 2011. *American Society of Health-System Pharmacists*. 1707-1760.

Pereira, B., Sayegh, M., and P. Blake. 2007. "Principles of Hemodialysis and its Medications." *Chronic Kidney Disease, Dialysis, and Transplantation*. 3rd Ed. 307-340.

Trissels, L. 2010. *Handbook on Injectable Drugs*. American Society of Health-System Pharmacists. 1209-1301.

Kastrup and Erwin K, et al. Drugs Facts and Comparison (2013)

2012 Top 200 Branded Drugs by Retail Dollars. Drug Topics (2012). (Source: SDI/Verispan, VONA, full year 2012.)

U.S. Food and Drug Administration. www.fda.gov

Index

www.ingramcontent.com/pod-product-compliance
Lightning Source LLC
Chambersburg PA
CBHW030949180526
45163CB00002B/716